Rikiya Fujita, Hiroshi Takahashi (Eds.)

Gastrointestinal Cancer Atlas for Endoscopic Therapy

Rikiya Fujita, Hiroshi Takahashi (Eds.)

Gastrointestinal Cancer Atlas for Endoscopic Therapy

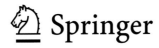 Springer

Rikiya Fujita, MD, DMSc, FACG
Consultant, Department of Endoscopy
The Cancer Institute Hospital of JFCR, Tokyo, Japan
Professor Emeritus, Showa University, Tokyo, Japan

Hiroshi Takahashi, MD, PhD
Director, Cancer Screening Center
The Cancer Institute Hospital of JFCR, Tokyo, Japan

Library of Congress Control Number: 2008942063

ISBN 978-4-431-88164-3 Springer Tokyo Berlin Heidelberg New York
e-ISBN 978-4-431-88166-7

Springer is a part of Springer Science+Business Media
springer.com

© Springer 2009

Printed in Japan
Typesetting: SNP Best-set Typesetter Ltd., Hong Kong
Printing and binding: Nikkei Printing Inc., Tokyo
Printed on acid-free paper

Preface

Early gastric cancer is routinely diagnosed and now accounts for 70% of all gastric cancers detected at the Ariake Hospital Cancer Institute. The same is true for early diagnosis of colorectal and esophageal cancers. The aim of this book is to introduce techniques for the diagnosis of early cancer, in particular, cancers of less than 5 mm in diameter, referred to as "minute cancer." These cancers can all be treated endoscopically.

The techniques of endoscopic mucosal resection (EMR) and endoscopic submucosal dissection (ESD), developed in Japan, have attracted international attention and have been adopted for live demonstrations at medical meetings. Although these activities are to be welcomed, case presentations on site are often difficult, because early and minute cancer cases are rarely detected under these circumstances. While detection of early cancer is indispensable for demonstration of these cutting-edge techniques, the introduction of diagnostics and supplementary diagnostics to support them are necessary.

To date, there have been rather few presentations using chromoscopy at international meetings except for those performed by Japanese, but it is encouraging that chromoscopy is becoming more generally employed and chromoscopic images can be presented worldwide. Recently, diagnostics employing computer image processing technologies, such as NBI (narrow band imaging, by Olympus) and FICE (Fuji intelligent color enhancement, by Fujinon), have been applied to facilitate this process.

It is believed that early cancer presents as a lesion and precedes advanced cancer. The fact that endoscopy is rarely indicated in cases of early cancer, which is generally asymptomatic, is a factor delaying diagnosis and complicating the situation. It is therefore important to suspect early cancer and obtain evidence of a lesion in "what is already seen" at the stage of detection.

Who sees with his/her eye believes with his/her heart.

For accurate diagnosis of gastrointestinal early cancer, it is also necessary to gather information on the morphological classification of minute and early cancers and to acquire experience in observing and assessing them. Inexperience may lead to misdiagnosis, even when a lesion is clearly present. Type 0-I, 0-IIa, and 0-IIb cancers may be misclassified as chronic gastritis or benign polyps, and type 0-IIc cancer as erosion or ulcer scarring. If no biopsy is taken, such early cancers can be overlooked.

We have experienced these kinds of difficulties when teaching physicians in foreign countries. Factors making detection of early cancer even more difficult derive from the traditional criteria of pathological diagnosis being used. Although there is little notable difference in the standards of biopsy-based pathological diagnosis in Japan, this is not the case in all countries, and there often seems to be a large discrepancy between cancer and dysplasia assessment elsewhere (see *Early Cancer of the Gastrointestinal Tract*, edited by Fujita, Jass, Kaminishi, and Schlemper; Springer, 2006). Readers may refer to the literature on the Paris classification in R. Lambert et al.: The Paris endoscopic classification of superficial neoplastic lesions: esophagus, stomach and colon. Gastrointest Endosc 2003:58 (suppl 6) 3–43.

It is delightful to have the opportunity to publish this book, and we are proud of our colleagues at the Cancer Institute of Ariake Hospital for their efforts in helping to write it. We strongly recommend that gastroenterologists engaged in endoscopic treatment read this book. We hope that diagnostics of minute and early cancer will prevail worldwide and contribute to the welfare of humankind.

Rikiya Fujita, MD, DMSc, FACG
Consultant, Department of Endoscopy
The Cancer Institute Hospital of JFCR, Tokyo, Japan
Professor Emeritus, Showa University, Tokyo, Japan

Contents

List of Contributors

Chino, Akiko (p. 110)
Gastroenterology Center, The Cancer Institute Hospital of JFCR, Tokyo, Japan

Fujisaki, Junko (p. 31, 95)
Department of Endoscopy, The Cancer Institute Hospital of JFCR, Tokyo, Japan

Fujisaki, Tadashi (p. 66, 68, 70)
Tokyo Metropolitan Tama Cancer Detection Center

Fumizono, Yutaka (p. 124)
Gastroenterology Center, The Cancer Institute Hospital of JFCR, Tokyo, Japan

Funatsu, Yasuhiro (p. 116)
Department of Endoscopy, The Cancer Institute Hospital of JFCR, Tokyo, Japan

Hayashi, Yuko (p. 72, 74, 76, 78, 80)
Gastroenterology Center, The Cancer Institute Hospital of JFCR, Tokyo, Japan

Hibiki, Taro (p. 118)
Department of Endoscopy, The Cancer Institute Hospital of JFCR, Tokyo, Japan

Hirasawa, Toshiaki (p. 86, 93)
Gastroenterology Center, The Cancer Institute Hospital of JFCR, Tokyo, Japan

Igarashi, Masahiro (p. 99)
Department of Endoscopy, The Cancer Institute Hospital of JFCR, Tokyo, Japan

Ishiyama, Akiyoshi (p. 9, 11, 13, 120)
Gastroenterology Center, The Cancer Institute Hospital of JFCR, Tokyo, Japan

Kishihara, Teruhito (p. 126)
Department of Endoscopy, The Cancer Institute Hospital of JFCR, Tokyo, Japan

Kuraoka, Kensuke (p. 46, 48, 54, 95)
Gastroenterology Center, The Cancer Institute Hospital of JFCR, Tokyo, Japan

Ogawa, Taishi (p. 113)
Department of Endoscopy, The Cancer Institute Hospital of JFCR, Tokyo, Japan

Okawa, Nobuhiko (p. 130)
Department of Endoscopy, The Cancer Institute Hospital of JFCR, Tokyo, Japan

Takahashi, Hiroshi (p. 21)
Cancer Screening Center, The Cancer Institute Hospital of JFCR, Tokyo, Japan

Tatewaki, Makoto (p. 56, 58, 60)
Tokyo Midtown Clinic, Tokyo, Japan

Tsuchida, Tomohiro (p. 3, 7, 15, 17)
Gastroenterology Center, The Cancer Institute Hospital of JFCR, Tokyo, Japan

Ueki, Nobue (p. 42, 44, 52)
Department of Endoscopy, The Cancer Institute Hospital of JFCR, Tokyo, Japan

Ukawa, Kunio (p. 72, 74, 76, 78, 80)
Cancer Screening Center, The Cancer Institute Hospital of JFCR, Tokyo, Japan

Uragami, Naoyuki (p. 105)
Gastroenterology Center, The Cancer Institute Hospital of JFCR, Tokyo, Japan

Yamamoto, Yorimasa (p. 36, 82, 84, 91)
Gastroenterology Center, The Cancer Institute Hospital of JFCR, Tokyo, Japan

Yoshimoto, Kazuhito (p. 50, 62, 64)
Gastroenterology Center, The Cancer Institute Hospital of JFCR, Tokyo, Japan

Keys to Diagnosis of Small and Minute Esophageal Cancer Including Diagnosis by Magnifying Endoscopy with Narrow Band Imaging

Tomohiro Tsuchida

Introduction

With the advent of endoscopic therapy, the treatment of superficial-type esophageal cancer has greatly changed. Even when this cancer is detected at an early stage, surgery, chemotherapy, or radiotherapy is required. For diagnosis of esophageal cancer in the early stages, it is necessary to enhance the conventional endoscopic examination through the use of esophageal iodine staining and narrow band imaging in patients at high risk of esophageal cancer. These high-risk patients include 1) men with smoking habits and/or excessive alcohol consumption, in particular those who exhibit alcohol-induced flushing; 2) patients with head and neck cancer; 3) patients with melanosis observed by upper gastrointestinal endoscopy; and 4) patients with a personal or family history of cancer.

Endoscopic Evaluation of Esophageal Squamous Cell Carcinoma

Routine Examination

Small superficial esophageal cancers show little surface irregularity, and most of these cancers can be detected by a mucosal color change. It is important to evaluate the color change by controlling air insufflation and desufflation during routine endoscopic examination. Under conditions in which the esophageal mucosa is extended by air insufflation, detecting a slightly reddish change is difficult. It is necessary to pay close attention to the pattern of the vascular network in the extended mucosa because vascular disruption suggests the presence of a lesion.

Iodine Staining

Upon iodine staining, normal esophageal mucosa appears brown, whereas abnormal mucosa is visualized as an unstained region. However, not only esophageal cancer

Fujita, Takahashi (Eds.), *Gastrointestinal Cancer Atlas for Endoscopic Therapy*, DOI: 10.1007/978-4-431-88166-7_1
© Springer

but also inflammatory changes (e.g., esophagitis) are observed as unstained regions. In high-risk groups, multiple unstained regions are often detected, and it is difficult to differentiate esophageal cancer from other abnormalities. In such cases, it is helpful to employ the "pink color sign" as a hallmark (1): Several minutes after spraying the iodine solution, a pink area appears in the unstained region. This color change is considered to be a positive "pink color sign," indicating that this area of the tissue is likely to be cancerous.

Narrow Band Imaging Endoscopy

Esophageal cancer is visualized as a brownish area by narrow band imaging (NBI), which, like iodine staining, allows early detection of cancerous regions. Furthermore, it has become possible to differentiate benign lesions from malignant ones by combining magnifying endoscopy with NBI to visualize microvasculature patterns in the mucosa (2). Fine, linear vessels are apparent in normal mucosa, whereas large, irregular vessels are observed in cancerous mucosa (Fig. 1). When a cancerous vascular pattern is detected, the lesion is later diagnosed as esophageal cancer in about 80% of endoscopic resections, even when the original diagnosis (at biopsy) was esophageal dysplasia.

Endoscopic Evaluation of Barrett's Esophagus and Barrett's Esophageal Cancer

In most cases, Barrett's esophagus stems from reflux esophagitis and is composed of the columnar epithelial metaplasia of squamous epithelial cells in the distal esophagus. Esophageal adenocarcinoma frequently occurs in the esophageal mucosa affected by Barrett's esophagus. Therefore, attention has been drawn to new techniques for monitoring Barrett's esophagus endoscopically, with the aim of early detection of Barrett's esophageal adenocarcinoma. The combination of magnifying endoscopy with the NBI technique has enabled endoscopic diagnosis by clear visualization of minute networks and capillary patterns in the mucosa (3).

Endoscopic Findings of Barrett's Esophageal Cancer

Dysplasia and early cancer resulting from Barrett's esophagus produce few macroscopic changes, making an endoscopic diagnosis difficult. If the lower esophagus is contracted, observation of the esophagocardiac junction (ECJ) itself is sometimes difficult; however, the area can be stretched sufficiently via deep inhalation by the patient and insufflation with air via the endoscope. It is important to observe the surface mucosal irregularity and color changes with caution.

For an endoscopic diagnosis, it is necessary to look carefully for any mucosal irregularity and color changes at the ECJ. When even a small change is observed, it

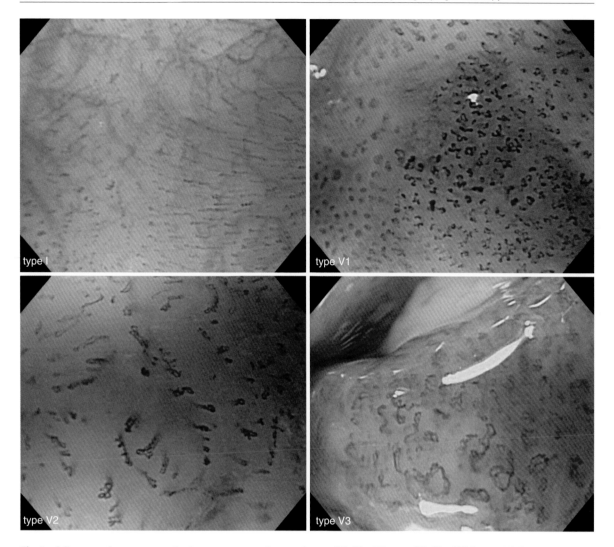

Fig. 1. Microvasculature patterns in the mucosa: *type I*, normal; *type VI*, T1a-EP; *type V2*, T1a-LPM; *type V3*, T1a-MM

is best to use staining and magnification in combination with NBI. Endoscopic observation with NBI reveals that the mucosal microvasculature becomes more obscure and abnormal vasculature becomes more conspicuous in cases of Barrett's esophageal adenocarcinoma compared to the vascular patterns observed in Barrett' esophagus. Similar to the vascular patterns observed in early gastric cancer (4) reticular, elliptical, and swirling vascular patterns, as well as a mixture of these patterns, can be observed (5).

References

1. Yokoyama A, Omori T, Yokoyama T (2007) Risk appraisal and endoscopic screening fir esophageal squamous cell carcinoma in Japanese populations. Esophagus 4:135–143
2. Inoue H, Honda T, Yoshida T, et al (1997) Ultra-high magnification endoscopic observation of carcinoma in situ of the esophagus. Dig Endosc 9:16–18

3. Goda K, Tajiri H, Nakayoshi T, et al (2004) Clinical significance of magnifying endoscopy combined with the narrow band imaging system for Barrett's esophagus. Stomach Intestine 39:1297–1307
4. Fujisaki J, Saito M, Yamamoto Y, et al (2006) Diagnosis of minute early gastric cancer using magnified endoscopy—especially using magnified narrow band imaging. Gastroenterol Endosc 48:1470–1479
5. Tsuchida T, Kuraoka S, Watanabe T, et al (2006) Usefulness of magnified narrow-band imaging (NBI) in diagnosing Barrett's esophageal adenocarcinoma. Clin Gastroenterol 9:45–49

Case 1

59-year-old man superficial esophageal cancer, 0-IIc, 8-mm squamous cell carcinoma.

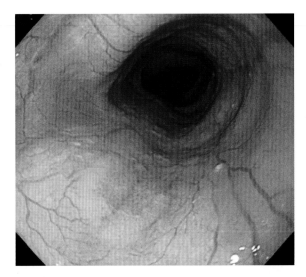

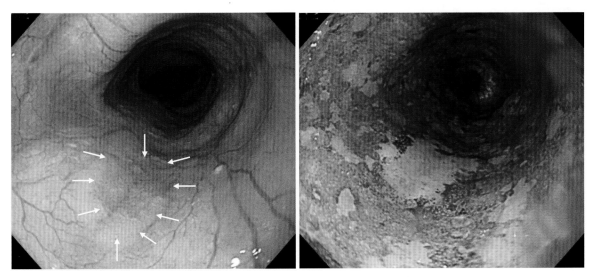

Fig. 1. Endoscopic diagnosis and findings
Routine observation: The lesion exhibited a mildly reddish depression without granular irregularity, but mucosal extension was preserved. Disruption of branch-like blood vessels was visualized (*arrows*)
Iodine staining: Note the multiple unstained areas. The lesion was seen as an 8-mm area that was unstained with iodine and located exactly at the reddish mucosa

Fujita, Takahashi (Eds.), *Gastrointestinal Cancer Atlas for Endoscopic Therapy*, DOI: 10.1007/978-4-431-88166-7_2
© Springer

Diagnostic Points:

The lesion was easily recognized by observations with NBI and iodine staining. Mucosal redness with disrupted blood vessels is a finding that should never be overlooked by routine observation.

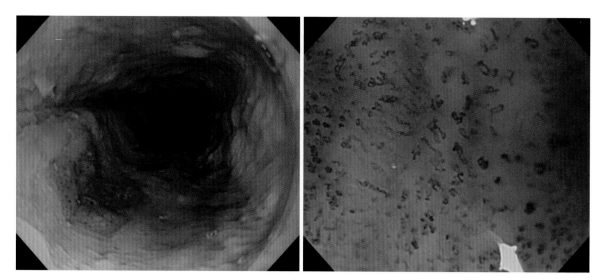

Fig. 2. Endoscopic diagnosis and findings
NBI: The lesion was visualized as a brownish area
Magnifying NBI: Type V vascular pattern is revealed

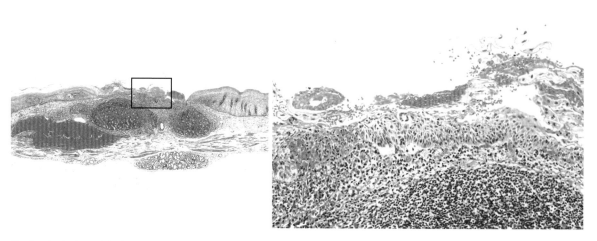

Fig. 3. *Pathological findings*: Squamous cell carcinoma, 0-IIc, T1a-EP, ly0, v0, HM0, VM0

Case 2

66-year-old man superficial esophageal cancer, 0-IIb, 6-mm squamous cell carcinoma.

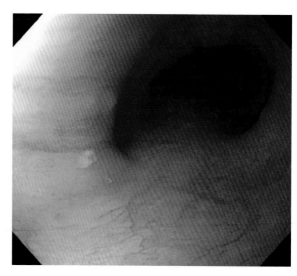

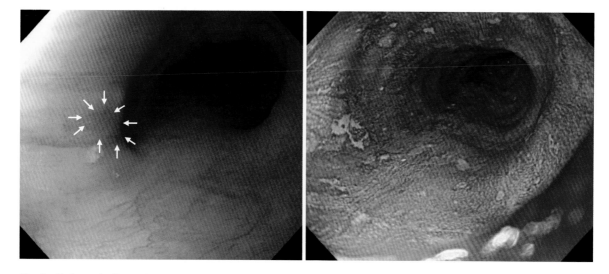

Fig. 1. Endoscopic diagnosis and findings
Routine observation: A 6-mm area with mild redness was observed (*arrows*). There was no mucosal irregularity. In terms of invasion depth, T1a-EP cancer was suspected
Iodine staining: There was an area unstained with iodine that corresponded to the site of a reddish depression seen by routine observation. The site was positive for the pink color sign

Diagnostic Points:

Metachronous multiple lesions were detected during the follow-up after endoscopic resection of a superficial-type esophageal cancer. It is important to pay close attention to the presence of metachronous multiple lesions. The finding of a positive pink color sign can help diagnose a small lesion.

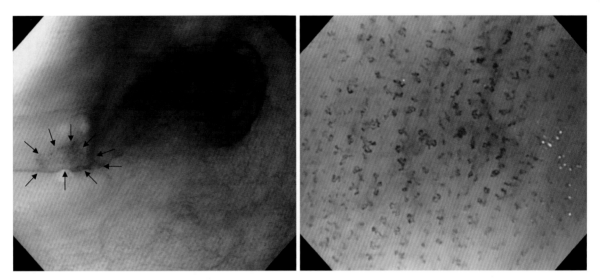

Fig. 2. Endoscopic diagnosis and findings
NBI: The lesion was visualized as a brownish area (*arrows*) that corresponded to the site of a reddish depression seen by routine observation
Magnifying NBI: Type V1 vascular pattern was revealed

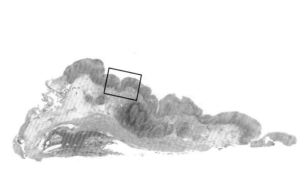
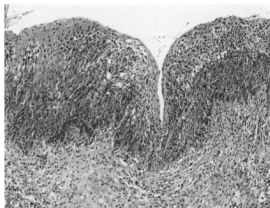

Fig. 3. *Pathological findings*: Squamous cell carcinoma, 0-IIb, T1a-EP, ly0, v0, HM0, VM0

Case 3

70-year-old man superficial esophageal cancer, 0-IIc,
6-mm squamous cell carcinoma.

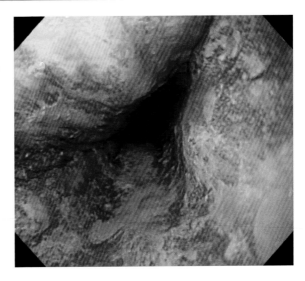

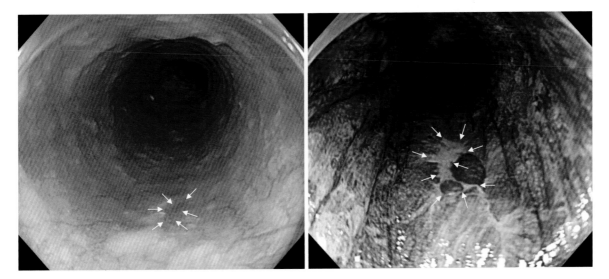

Fig. 1. Endoscopic diagnosis and findings
Routine observation: An area unstained with iodine extended longitudinally from the lower esophagus (*arrows*). Reexamination after administration of a proton pump inhibitor (PPI) revealed a mildly reddish area 6 mm in diameter at the same region
Iodine staining: An area unstained with iodine (*arrows*) was observed at exactly the same site of a reddish depression observed by routine observation. The site was positive for the pink color sign

Diagnostic Points:

Background inflammation was severe, and the margin was unclear. After PPI administration, inflammation subsided and the margin became clearer. A positive pink color sign would help diagnose the margin of the lesion.

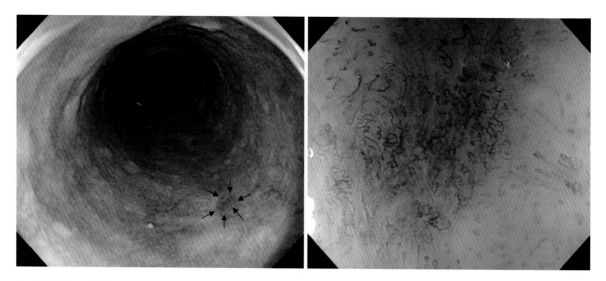

Fig. 2. Endoscopic diagnosis and findings
NBI: The lesion was visualized as a brownish area corresponding to the site of the reddish depression detected by routine observation
Magnifying NBI: Note that blood vessels are thin and extended owing to inflammation (*arrows*); a V3 vascular pattern was observed in part. Invasion depth TIb-MM to SM1 was suspected

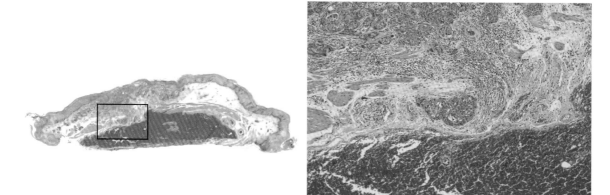

Fig. 3. *Pathological findings*: Squamous cell carcinoma, 0-IIc, T1b-SM (127 μm), ly0, v0, HM0, VM0

Case 4

70-year-old man superficial esophageal cancer, 0-IIc, 8-mm squamous cell carcinoma.

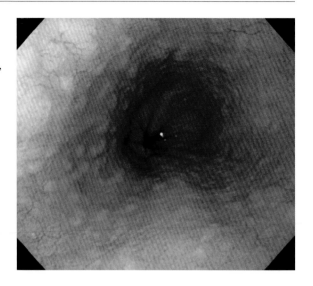

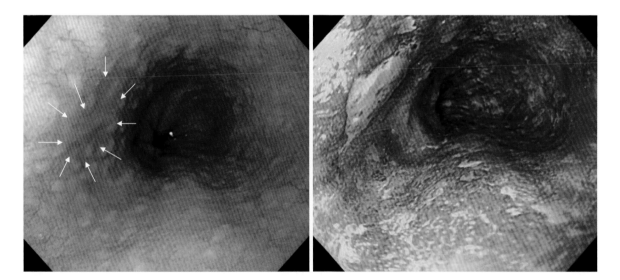

Fig. 1. Endoscopic diagnosis and findings
Routine observation: A mildly reddish area of about 8 mm was seen (*arrows*). Given the absence of evident granular changes at the redness, an invasion depth T1a-EP cancer was suspected
Iodine staining: An area unstained with iodine was observed at the site of the redness seen by routine observation

Diagnostic Points:

Iodine-unstained areas were scattered, but a positive pink color sign was recognized only at this site, which would help lead to the diagnosis.

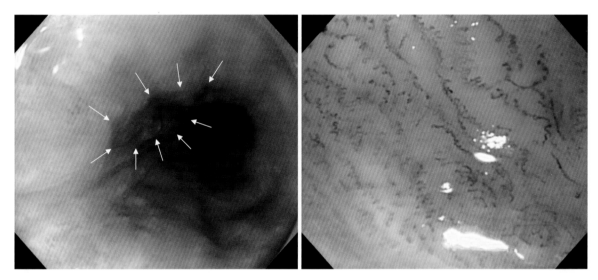

Fig. 2. Endoscopic diagnosis and findings
NBI: The lesion was visualized as a brownish area (*arrows*) at the site of the redness detected by routine observation
Magnifying NBI: Type VI vascular pattern was revealed

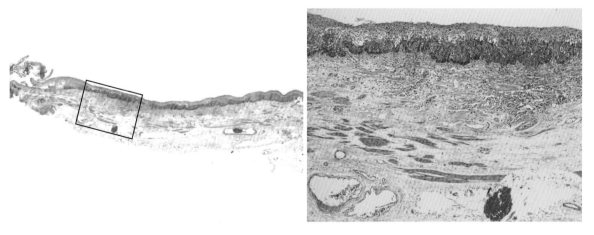

Fig. 3. *Pathological findings*: Squamous cell carcinoma, 0-IIc, T1a-LPM, ly0, v0, HM0, VM0

Case 5

71-year-old man superficial esophageal cancer, 0-IIb, 5-mm squamous cell carcinoma.

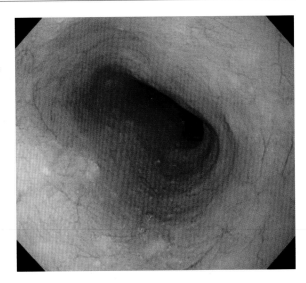

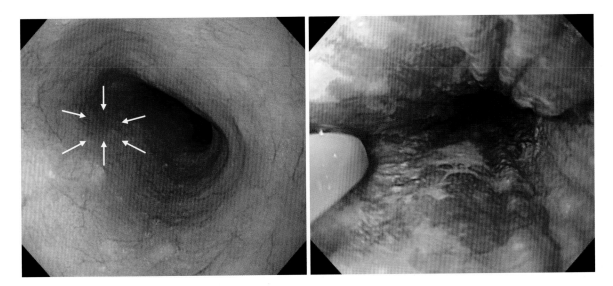

Fig. 1. Endoscopic diagnosis and findings
Routine observation: The lesion (*arrows*) was difficult to detect by routine observation
Iodine staining: The lesion was seen as an area unstained with iodine and with a positive pink color sign

Diagnostic Points:

The iodine-unstained area with a positive pink color sign and a type V vascular pattern are suggestive of malignancy.

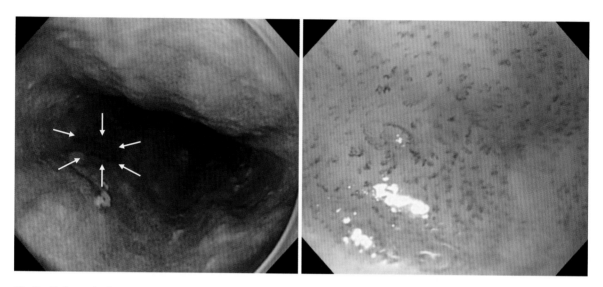

Fig. 2. Endoscopic diagnosis and findings
NBI: The lesion was visualized as a brownish area (*arrows*)
Magnifying NBI: Type V vascular pattern was revealed

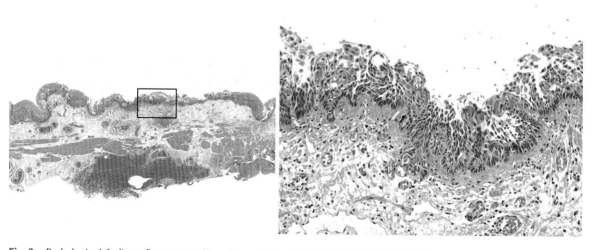

Fig. 3. *Pathological findings*: Squamous cell carcinoma, 0-IIc, T1a-LPM, ly0, v0, HM0, VM0

Case 6

71-year-old man Barrett's esophageal cancer, 0-IIc, 5-mm adenocarcinoma (tub 1).

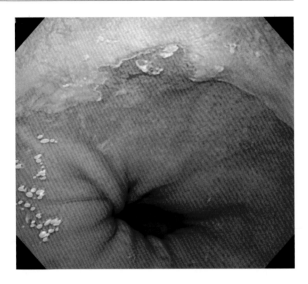

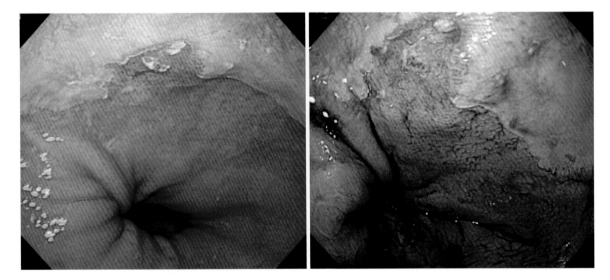

Fig. 1. Endoscopic diagnosis and findings

Routine observation: There was a reddish depression protruding from the squamous-columnar junction (SCJ) to the squamous cell epithelium in the shape of a tongue. Although lower esophageal palisade vessels were unclear, the SCJ appeared irregular; and the presence of short-segment Barrett's esophagus (SSBE) was suspected

Indigo carmine staining: Depression of the lesion became clearer. There was no surface irregularity at the depression

Diagnostic Point:

It is necessary to observe carefully the reddish mucosa at the SCJ. In particular, when SSBE is present, detecting a change in mucosal structure and abnormal blood vessels by magnifying NBI would help with the diagnosis.

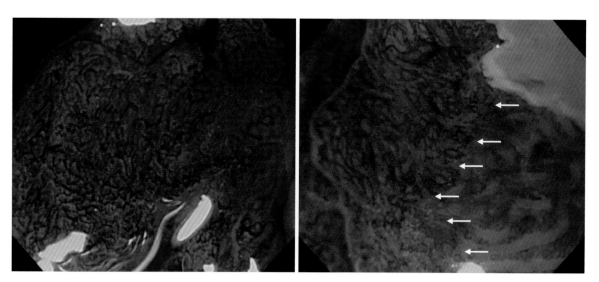

Fig. 2. Endoscopic diagnosis and findings
Magnifying NBI: Reticular vascular pattern was observed at the depression, strongly suggesting malignancy
Magnifying NBI: A change in mucosal structure at the margin of the depression was revealed, which better demarcated the boundary

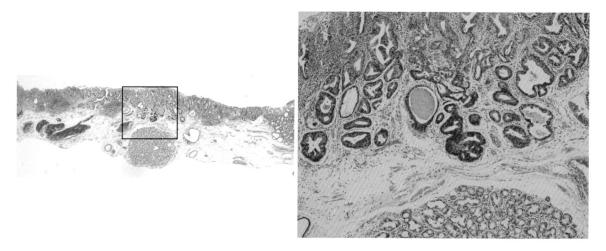

Fig. 3. *Pathohistological findings*: Adenocarcinoma (tub 1), M, ly0, v0, HM0, VM0

Part II

Stomach

Endoscopic Diagnosis of Early Small and Minute Gastric Cancer

Hiroshi Takahashi

Introduction

Needless to say, detecting a lesion of the smallest size possible has a great beneficial impact on decisions regarding subsequent treatment strategy. In particular, detecting a lesion at the stage that allows endoscopic treatment is a key goal of the endoscopist. During endoscopic examinations, attention should be paid to the following points.

- Comfortable endoscopy facilitates clinical follow-up of patients.
- Complete removal of mucus is fundamental to endoscopy.
- Conforming to the standards of observation helps avoid overlooking irregularities.
- Changing the air amount and patient position depending on the situation is important.
- Constant attention to even minimal findings is needed.
- Chromoendoscopy requires ingenuity.
- Conventional diagnostic approaches can produce poor results.

These seven Cs are critical to the success of endoscopic diagnosis.

It is necessary to optimize the conditions under which endoscopic diagnosis is performed by fine-tuning the examination techniques. These conditions range from the diagnostic capability of the examination method to the status of the patient.

In particular, it is extremely useful during the examination always to pay close attention to mucosal changes instead of focusing on a single lesion (Figs. 1, 2). Furthermore, for the detection of minute lesions, it is helpful to use the dye-spraying technique effectively (Figs. 3, 4).

Findings of Minute Gastric Cancer

Endoscopic findings of minute gastric cancer (≤5 mm in diameter) and small gastric cancer (>5 to ≤10 mm) observed in our institution were examined to clarify where attention was especially needed to detect a small lesion.

Fujita, Takahashi (Eds.), *Gastrointestinal Cancer Atlas for Endoscopic Therapy*, DOI: 10.1007/978-4-431-88166-7_3
© Springer

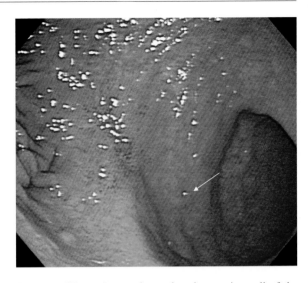

Fig. 1. *Routine observation*: An ulcer scar (S1 stage) was observed at the anterior wall of the mid-body of the stomach accompanied by a minute depression at the anal side (*arrow*)

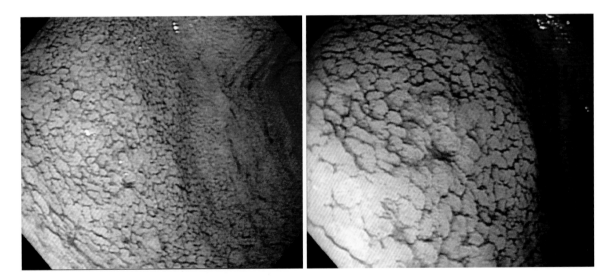

Fig. 2. *Indigo carmine spraying*: Dye spraying more clearly visualized the depression and made it easier to diagnose the presence of the lesion

Patient Characteristics

A total of 118 patients with minute gastric cancers and 114 patients with small gastric cancers detected by endoscopy were enrolled in this study. The average age of the patients was 68.8 years, and there were 181 men and 51 women.

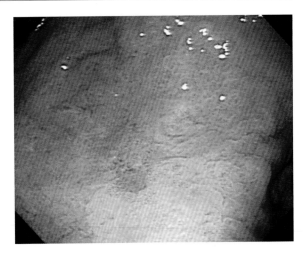

Fig. 3. *Routine observation*: A reddish depressive lesion was observed at the greater curvature of the fornix

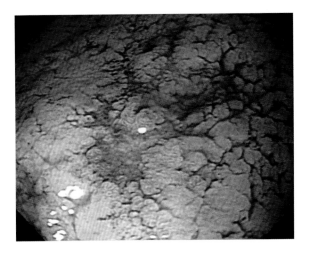

Fig. 4. *Indigo carmine spraying*: Dye spraying more clearly visualized the depression and made it easier to diagnose the presence of the lesion

Lesions

Whether the gastric cancer lesions were solitary or multiple was examined. Minute cancer was observed as solitary in 69 cases (58%) and multiple in 49 cases (42%). On the other hand, small cancer was found to be solitary in 79 cases (69%) and multiple in 35 cases (31%) (Table 1). In terms of the background of minute and small cancers, it was noteworthy that multiple lesions were observed frequently. Gastric cancer was concurrently present or had been resected in the past (history of surgical or endoscopic resection) in 42% of minute gastric cancer cases and 31% of small gastric cancer cases. Kato reported that solitary and multiple gastric cancers were found in 6.3% and 18.5%, respectively, of 1716 surgically resected stomachs that were thin-sliced thoroughly for pathological examinations (1). These results suggest that detailed examinations are desirable in patients with a past history of gastric cancer.

Table 1. Characteristics of subjects with gastric cancer. *MGC*, minute gastric cancer; *SGC*, small gastric cancer

MGC (≤5 mm) n = 118	N = 232	n = 114 SGC (6–10 mm)
Age		
68.1 years	68.8 years	69.5 years
Sex		
M:F	M:F	M:F
93:25	181:51	88:26
Number of lesions		
Solitary:multiple	Solitary:multiple	Solitary:multiple
69:49	148:84	79:35

Table 2. Location of minute gastric cancers (*n* = 118). *AW*, anterior wall; *PW*, posterior wall; *LC*, lesser curvature; *GC*, greater curvature. Numbers in parentheses are the number of undifferentiated adenocarcinomas

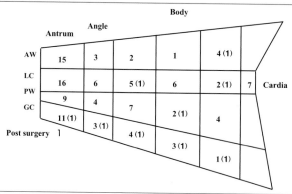

Localization

Minute gastric cancers were found predominantly in the antrum, with the numbers detected at the angle and body being comparable (Table 2). Undifferentiated cancer was found predominantly at the greater curvature of the gastric corpus (Table 2). Similar trends occurred for the location of the small gastric cancers, which were found most frequently in the antrum (Table 3).

Endoscopic Morphology and Pathohistological Diagnosis

The endoscopic morphology and pathohistological findings for the gastric cancers are summarized in Table 4. There were 118 minute gastric cancers with the following distribution.

- 0-IIa: 17 (differentiated adenocarcinomas, 17; undifferentiated adenocarcinoma, 0)
- 0-IIb: 3 (differentiated adenocarcinomas, 1; undifferentiated adenocarcinomas, 2)
- 0-IIc: 98 (differentiated adenocarcinomas, 89; undifferentiated adenocarcinomas, 9)

Table 3. Location of small gastric cancers ($n = 114$)

Table 4. Pathohistological findings for gastric cancers. *Diff*, differentiated adenocarcinoma; *Undiff*, undifferentiated adenocarcinoma

MGC (≤5 mm) n = 118	N = 232	n = 114 SGC (6–10 mm)
	0-I	1
	1	Diff.:1 Undiff.:O
	Diff.:1	
17	0-IIa	24
Diff.:17 Undiff.:O	41	Diff.:24 Undiff.:O
	Diff.:41 Undiff.:O	
3	0-IIb	2
Diff.:1 Undiff.:2	5	Diff.:1 Undiff.:1
	Diff.:2 Undiff.:3	
98	0-IIc	86
Diff.:89 Undiff.:9	184	Diff.:71 Undiff.:15
	Diff.:160 Undiff.:24	

There were 114 small gastric cancers, with the following distribution.

- 0-I: 1 (differentiated adenocarcinoma, 1; undifferentiated adenocarcinoma, 0)
- 0-IIa: 24 (differentiated adenocarcinomas, 24; undifferentiated adenocarcinoma, 0)
- 0-IIb: 2 (differentiated adenocarcinoma, 1; undifferentiated adenocarcinoma, 1)
- 0-IIc: 86 (differentiated adenocarcinomas, 71; undifferentiated adenocarcinomas, 15)

Characteristic Endoscopic Findings

0-I and 0-IIa Gastric Cancer

0-IIa Minute Gastric Cancer

There were 17 cases of 0-IIa minute gastric cancer (Table 5). Upon endoscopy, 13 of the 17 cases (76%) showed a pale color change compared with the adjacent

Table 5. Elevated-type early gastric cancer

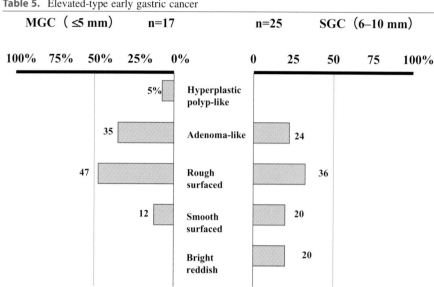

| MGC (≤5 mm) | n=17 | | n=25 | SGC (6–10 mm) |

mucosa. Six of them showed adenoma-like surface irregularity, but differentiation from adenoma was difficult based on the endoscopic findings. There were two cases without color changes, and hyperplastic polyp-like findings were observed in one case.

0-I and 0-IIa Small Gastric Cancer

The findings included 1 case of 0-I and 24 cases of 0-IIa small gastric cancer (Table 5). Upon endoscopy, in 12 of the 25 cases (48%), the lesion showed a pale color change compared with the adjacent mucosa. Six of them showed adenoma-like surface irregularity, but differentiation from adenoma was difficult based on endoscopic findings. No color change was observed in four cases, and reddish flat-elevated areas were found in four cases.

As noted in previous reports, because 0-I and 0-IIa gastric cancers were identified based on finding an elevated area with redness (similar to hyperplastic polyps) or a whitish lesion compared with the adjacent mucosa (as in cases of adenoma), it was difficult to differentiate these cancers.

0-IIb Gastric Cancer

0-IIb Minute Gastric Cancer

There were three cases of 0-IIb minute gastric cancer (Table 6). Qualitative endoscopic diagnosis was relatively difficult, and it was considered important to pay close attention to "brownish spots" and "heterogeneously reddish spots" for their detection. With regard to histology, two of the lesions were signet-ring cell carcinomas, and one was a well-differentiated adenocarcinoma. The endoscopic findings distin-

Table 6. Flat (IIb)-type early gastric cancer

MGC (≤5 mm) n = 3	n = 2 SGC (6–10 mm)
Diff. 1	Diff. 0
Reddish	
uneven mucosa	
Undiff. 2	Undiff. 2
Pale	Pale

guished between these two types of cancer in that well-differentiated adenocarci-noma was observed as "mild redness," whereas the two signet-ring cell carcinomas were visualized as "pale spots."

0-IIb Small Gastric Cancer

There were two cases of 0-IIb small gastric cancer (Table 6). Qualitative endoscopic diagnosis was relatively difficult, and it was considered important to pay close attention to "pale spots" and "variegated reddish spots" for their detection. With regard to histology, one lesion was signet-ring cell carcinoma and one was well-differentiated adenocarcinoma. The endoscopic findings distinguished between these two types of cancer in that well-differentiated adenocarcinoma was observed as "mild redness," whereas the one case of signet-ring cell carcinoma was visualized as "pale spots."

As for the diagnosis of minute 0-IIb gastric cancer, there was no key point other than paying attention to the color change. In other words, it was a lesion recognized as a reddish or pale spot. Thus, undifferentiated cancer was characterized by pale spots.

0-IIc Minute Gastric Cancer

0-IIc Minute Gastric Cancer

The 98 cases of 0-IIc minute gastric cancer (89 differentiated, 9 undifferentiated) (Tables 7 and 8, respectively) showed a variety of forms with marked malignant findings, ranging from cases with an easy qualitative endoscopic diagnosis to those in which a qualitative diagnosis of detected lesions was difficult but possible. Furthermore, in some cases, it was difficult even to detect the presence of a lesion. Most of the lesions were characterized by "erosion," with solitary erosion being found in 77 cases (79%).

Endoscopic findings of 0-IIc minute gastric cancer depended on the histology. Differentiated cancer (Table 7) was associated with redness in 58 cases (59%), variegated color changes in 17 (19%), and no color change in 22 (24%). Encroachment, often a sign of malignancy, was observed in only 34 cases (38%); however, when irregularity of the depressed surface was taken into account, malignant findings were confirmed in 79%. Marginal swelling was observed in 48 cases (51%). In contrast, undifferentiated adenocarcinoma (Table 8) was a pale color in all cases, with both encroachment and marginal swelling found in only one case.

Table 7. Depressed (IIc)-type early gastric cancer (differentiated adenocarcinoma)

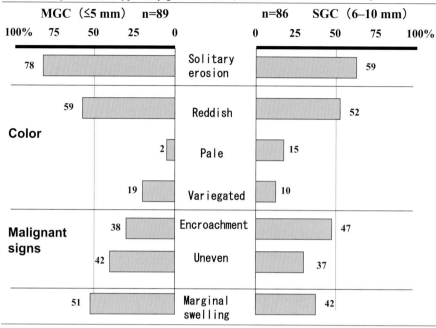

Table 8. Depresssed (IIc)-type early gastric cancer (undifferentiated adenocarcinoma)

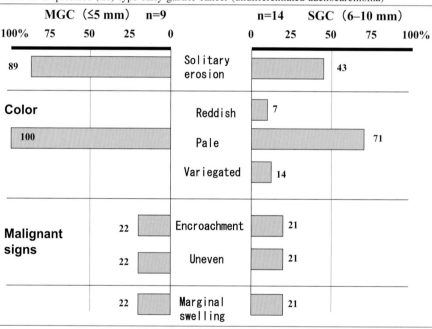

0-IIc Small Gastric Cancer

There were 100 cases of 0-IIc small gastric cancer (86 differentiated, 14 undifferenti-ated) (Tables 7 and 8, respectively). Endoscopic findings of 0-IIc small gastric cancer depended on the histology. Differentiated cancer ($n = 86$) was associated with redness in 44 cases (52%), pale in 13 (15%), and variegated color changes in 7 (8%). Encroachment, often a sign of malignancy, was observed in 40 cases (47%). When irregularity of the depressed surface was taken into account, malignant findings were confirmed in 84%. In addition, marginal swelling was found in 36 cases (42%). In contrast, all undifferentiated cancer cases (14 cases) had a pale brownish color, with both encroachment and marginal swelling being found in only 3 cases.

Regarding the diagnosis of 0-IIc early gastric cancer, lesions accompanied by marked encroachment were easy to diagnose qualitatively. However, in minute gastric cancers, malignant findings such as "abrupt ending of the fold," "encroachment of the border," and "irregularity of the depressed surface" were rarely observed, making qualitative endoscopic diagnosis difficult.

The results of the current study suggest that both encroachment at the margin and irregularity of the depressed surface were each observed in about 40% of cases, but one or the other was observed in about 80% of the cases, which indicates that observing the margin and depressed surface of the lesion in detail enables a diagnosis.

As to the size of the depression and depth of minute gastric cancer, a lesion of ≥4 mm with a deep depression allows detection of malignant findings with relative ease, making qualitative endoscopic diagnosis possible. When the lesion is smaller and the depression shallow, as we previously reported, attention should be paid not to conventional malignant hallmarks but, rather, to variegated color changes and asteroid redness, which are suggestive of cancer (2). Therefore, it would be possible to detect minute gastric cancer more frequently by routine endoscopy if the examination is performed more carefully.

Conclusion

The major aim of medical screening for gastric cancer is to decrease disease mortality. Early detection of gastric cancer allows the option of less invasive endoscopic treatment as an alternative to conventional surgery. Because endoscopic treatment greatly benefits the patients' quality of life, endoscopists should aim to diagnose a lesion at the endoscopically treatable stage. From this point of view, we investigated the factors critical to the detection of endoscopically resectable lesions.

In providing information for diagnosis, endoscopic examinations offer the advantage of visualizing the color changes of the lesions. These color changes are key indicators of the diagnosis of flat-type lesions typical of 0-IIb early gastric cancer—with redness, pale, and variegated color changes serving as important findings. In fact, in case of a minute gastric cancer, the color changes are key findings that allow identification of the lesion. It is therefore necessary to pay attention not only to morphological changes (e.g., depression, elevation) but to color changes as well, as these key mucosal alterations allow a diagnosis of minute gastric cancer.

We endeavor to detect superficial, small, and minute gastric cancer on the basis of these findings. With this objective in mind, it is essential for the endoscopist to optimize observation conditions by fine-tuning the examination techniques. These conditions range from the diagnostic limitations of the examination method to the status of the patient.

References

1. Kato Y (1990) A pathologist's recommendation to endoscopists regarding microcarcinoma of the stomach. Endosc Dig 3:287–290
2. Takahashi H, Kirihara K, Yamada M, et al (1998) Evaluation of the endoscopic features of minute gastric cancer. Stomach Intestine 33:609–616

Diagnosis of Minute Gastric Cancer by Narrow Band Imaging

Junko Fujisaki

Introduction

Narrow band imaging (NBI) is a new electronic endoscopy system ideally suited to the observation of surface structures, including capillaries. With NBI, short-wavelength light radiated through a narrow band filter is strongly absorbed by hemoglobin, thereby allowing surface vascular structures to be distinctly visualized (1).

Histology and NBI Evaluation of Surface Structure in Early Gastric Cancer

Narrow band imaging can visualize surface morphology, mostly manifested as mucosal microvascular patterns. Surface vascular patterns are roughly divided into two types that are associated with histological characteristics: well-differentiated and undifferentiated adenocarcinoma (2).

Well-Differentiated Adenocarcinoma

The surface vascular patterns of typical depressed-type early gastric cancer and well-differentiated adenocarcinoma show regularly arranged reticular vascular patterns (Fig. 1a). Histopathology has revealed that capillaries are present between regularly arranged cancer glands, and these blood vessels stain positive for CD34 (Fig. 1b).

Undifferentiated Adenocarcinoma

Undifferentiated adenocarcinoma is a typical depressed-type early gastric cancer whose histology shows irregular surface vascular patterns that can be visualized by

Fujita, Takahashi (Eds.), *Gastrointestinal Cancer Atlas for Endoscopic Therapy*, DOI: 10.1007/978-4-431-88166-7_4
© Springer

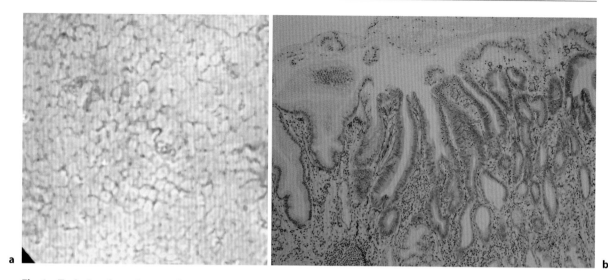

Fig. 1. Typical surface microvascular patterns and histology of well-differentiated adenocarcinoma
a Narrow band imaging (NBI) showed a fine reticular pattern
b Histology revealed regularly arranged capillaries staining positive for CD34 between cancer glands with mild structural irregularity in well-differentiated adenocarcinoma, reflecting the NBI findings

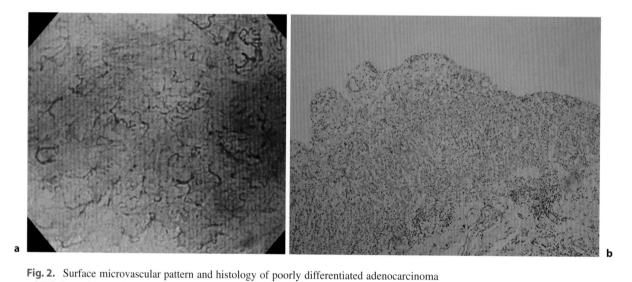

Fig. 2. Surface microvascular pattern and histology of poorly differentiated adenocarcinoma
a NBI showed irregular vascular patterns
b Histology revealed that each cancer cell was present scattered in the mucosa with abundant stroma. Capillaries were scattered at the surface in this poorly differentiated adenocarcinoma

NBI (Fig. 2a). The cancer cells are scattered, and spotty intervening blood vessels in the stroma are observed at the mucosal surface. Upon histopathological analysis, irregularly arranged blood vessels staining positive for CD34 are observed in the stroma of the mucosal surface, which reflect the irregular capillary images visualized by NBI (Fig. 2b).

Histology and NBI Findings in Minute Gastric Cancer

Well-Differentiated Adenocarcinoma

The well-differentiated 0-IIc lesion has been visualized at the posterior wall of the antrum by conventional endoscopy as well as by endoscopy after indigo carmine spraying (Fig. 3a,b). Figure 3c shows an image of such a case obtained by magnifying endoscopy with NBI. Fine reticular patterns were observed. Endoscopic submucosal dissection was carried out, and histology revealed a well-differentiated adenocarcinoma 3 mm in diameter (Fig. 3d). Cancer was identified only at the central depression. A high-power view of its histology is seen in Fig. 3e.

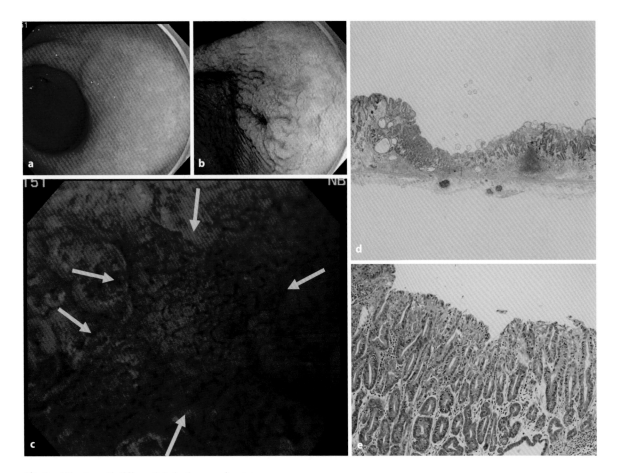

Fig. 3. Minute well-differentiated adenocarcinoma
a, b This 0-IIc early gastric cancer was located at the posterior wall of the antrum. Indigo carmine spraying clearly demarcated a depression that was 3 mm in diameter
c NBI showed a reticular vascular pattern (*arrows*)
d, e Histology revealed that the cancer was restricted to the depression and was diagnosed as well-differentiated adenocarcinoma

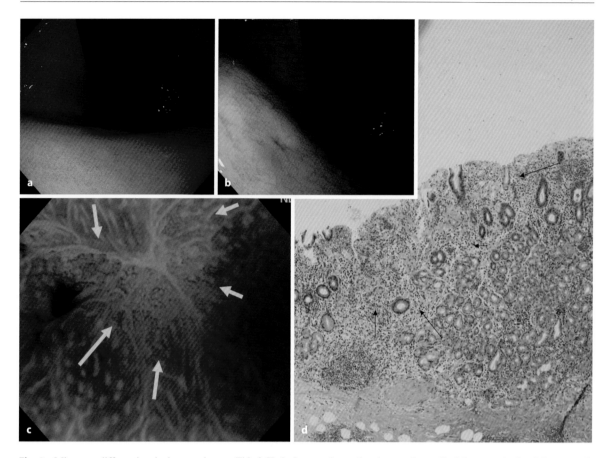

Fig. 4. Minute undifferentiated adenocarcinoma. This 0-IIc lesion was located at the anterior wall of the upper body of the stomach
a, **b** Conventional endoscopy showed a small discolored area, and indigo carmine spraying clearly demarcated a depression 3 mm in diameter
c NBI showed an irregular vascular pattern (*arrows*)
d Histology revealed signet-ring cell carcinoma

Undifferentiated Adenocarcinoma

The undifferentiated 0-IIc lesion is detected as a discolored area at the posterior wall of the mid-body of the stomach (Fig. 4a,b). In this case, biopsy led to the diagnosis of signet-ring cell carcinoma. Irregular vascular patterns were observed by NBI (Fig. 4c). Endoscopic mucosal resection was carried out, and pathology revealed a signet-ring cell carcinoma 3 mm in diameter, with the invasion depth limited to the mucosa (Fig. 4d).

Problems When Diagnosing Minute Early Gastric Cancer by NBI

Because NBI visualizes changes in surface structure, it is impossible to observe any irregular surface vascular patterns for signet-ring cell carcinomas that proliferate only at the regenerative zone or for cancers that develop in the deep, middle part of the mucosa, which is covered with regenerative and foveolar epithelium. Regarding minute cancers, it is sometimes impossible to identify typical vascular patterns after biopsy because the surface is covered with regenerative epithelium.

Importance of Diagnosing Minute Early Gastric Cancer by NBI

If minute early gastric cancer is suspected based on routine endoscopic observation, it can be confirmed when vascular patterns typical of cancer are observed at the surface by magnifying endoscopy with NBI. Similarly, if it is difficult to determine whether a lesion is caused by erosion or early gastric cancer, the lesion should be examined using NBI, which offers the advantage of avoiding biopsy when normal surface patterns are visualized.

Conclusion

In early gastric cancer, surface capillary patterns and minute surface structures exhibit characteristic features when visualized using magnifying endoscopy with NBI. With regard to the surface capillary patterns, well-differentiated adenocarcinoma and undifferentiated adenocarcinoma specifically show reticular and irregular vascular patterns, respectively. It is possible to diagnose minute gastric cancer before biopsy based on these NBI-visualized patterns.

References

1. Gono T, Yamazaki K, Doguchi N, et al (2003) Endoscopic observation of tissue by narrowband illumination. Optic Rev 10:211–215
2. Nakayoshi N, Tajiri H, Matsuda K, et al (2004) Magnifying endoscopy combined with narrow band imaging system for early gastric cancer: correlation of vascular pattern with histopathology (including video). Endoscopy 36:1080–1084

Endoscopic Treatment of Minute Gastric Cancer in Cases of a Disappearing-Cancer Biopsy

Yorimasa Yamamoto

Introduction

When diagnosing early gastric cancer by endoscopy, a lesion diameter of 3 mm has been thought to represent the lower limit of detection (1). In general, minute cancer is defined as a tumor ≤5 mm in diameter. Owing to the advances in endoscopic devices, it has become possible to diagnose gastric cancer preoperatively using magnifying endoscopy with narrow band imaging (NBI) (2), although a pathological diagnosis by biopsy is usually employed.

About 70% of minute gastric cancers detected preoperatively are macroscopically the depressed type. However, depressed-type small and minute gastric cancers may change morphologically after biopsy because of a decrease in the cancer volume due to the biopsy (3). The width of the biopsy forceps used for general endoscopic examinations is 6 mm when opened, so a biopsy can potentially remove most of the minute gastric cancer tissue.

Some minute gastric cancers are diagnosed by biopsy but cannot be visualized later when the cancer site is endoscopically reexamined to formulate the treatment strategy. In some of these cases, detailed exploration of the expected site of the lesion during surgical or endoscopic mucosal resection fails to locate the cancer. Such cancers may have been completely removed by the biopsy and are therefore termed "disappearing cancer" ("scratch cancer" in Japan) (4) (Figs. 1, 2).

When a lesion is followed up as a "disappearing cancer," however, it may be diagnosed as cancer with invasion to the submucosal (sm) layer, and careful follow-up should be undertaken (5).

The Problem of "Scratch Cancer"

The following issues can be raised concerning cancer disappearing after biopsy.

- Was the diagnosis of cancer at the time of the first biopsy accurate?
- Was the site detected as cancerous by the first biopsy the same site subsequently reexamined or treated?
- Was cancer indeed absent from the tissue that was surgically or endoscopically resected?

Fujita, Takahashi (Eds.), *Gastrointestinal Cancer Atlas for Endoscopic Therapy*, DOI: 10.1007/978-4-431-88166-7_5
© Springer

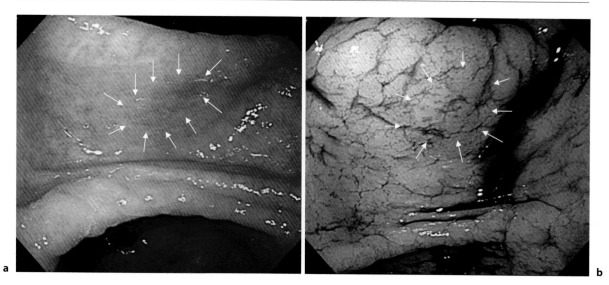

Fig. 1. a *Routine observation.* Vasculature was invisible, and a reddish area was visualized at the lesser curvature of the gastric angle (*arrows*). There was no distinct elevation or depression
b *Indigo carmine spraying.* Dye spraying revealed that the reddish area had an irregular depression at the center and mild elevations at the periphery (*arrows*). It resembled a type 0-IIc lesion (3 mm in diameter, peripheral reactive elevation), but encroachment at the margin was unclear

As to the first question, it is necessary, first, to confirm that the sample was not mistaken for another one. Second, the examiner must discuss the validity of the lesion's histological diagnosis as cancer with two or more pathologists before determining the treatment strategy (4).

With regard to the second question, when minute cancer is suspected based on the endoscopic findings of the first biopsy, it is necessary to record several images of the site in distant and close views under different air–volume conditions and to identify landmarks such as mucosal folds, ulcer scars, and xanthomas to establish the orientation more easily. It has been suggested that when minute cancer is suspected only part of it should be biopsied, with some left behind to avoid complete disappearance of the lesion (5). However, there is a high likelihood that minute cancer can become unidentifiable after the biopsy due to bleeding. Therefore, it may be necessary to collect a sample containing the entire lesion during the initial biopsy. In addition, incomplete biopsy (leaving part of the lesion in place) should be avoided because a small biopsy sample makes pathological diagnosis difficult; thus, the presence or absence of cancer may not be accurately diagnosed.

Sometimes minute cancer lacks the features suggestive of cancer at the first biopsy, and images that make identification of the lesion site difficult may be the only ones recorded. In such cases, endoscopy should be repeated as soon as possible, making sure to identify the erosion and scars associated with the initial biopsy, record images that allow quick orientation, and leave a mark adjacent to the lesion (injection of Indian ink) to enable confirmation of the site at the time of treatment (4).

When there are findings suggestive of minute cancer before a biopsy, a recently developed diagnostic technique, magnifying endoscopy, provides the option of detecting vascular patterns suggestive of malignancy and then immediately performing endoscopic resection without biopsy (4). This method can be used only when the patient's informed consent has been obtained in advance. The identification of

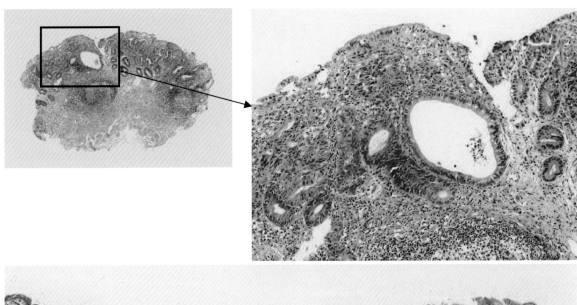

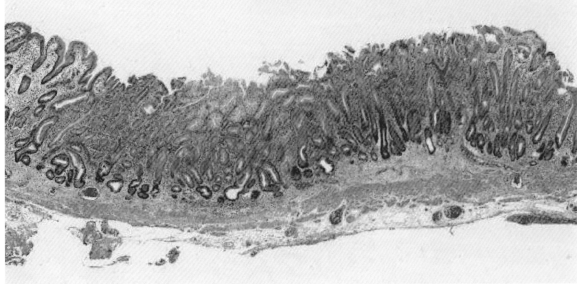

Fig. 2. a *Biopsy specimen*. Well-differentiated adenocarcinoma was observed, with swollen nuclei up to the mucosal surface and an irregular glandular structure
b *ESD specimen*. This endoscopic submucosal dissection (ESD) specimen failed to reveal cancer distinctly, and no cancer was observed in the specimen after additional thin slicing

vascular patterns specific for cancer by magnifying endoscopy combined with NBI has increased the diagnostic accuracy (2).

In terms of the third question, it has previously been reported that the disappearance of cancer after biopsy can be confirmed upon surgical resection (1), but less invasive endoscopic resection has increasingly been carried out (6, 7). Recently, endoscopic submucosal dissection (ESD) has been performed widely to treat early gastric cancer (8). By allowing resection of an entire area in one piece, this technique has enabled detailed pathological assessment of the resected specimen. When treating minute gastric cancer, so long as the lesion can be identified it can be treated by conventional endoscopic mucosal resection (EMR). However, when an entire cancer-

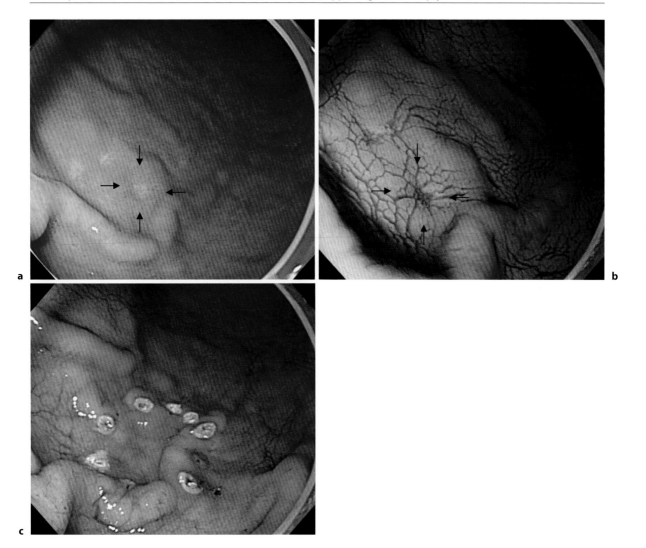

Fig. 3. a *Routine observation*. A discolored depression 3 mm in diameter was observed at the greater curvature of the lower body (*arrows*)
b *Indigo carmine spraying*. Indigo carmine spraying more clearly visualized the margin of the discolored depression (*arrows*). Signet-ring cell carcinoma (sig) was diagnosed by biopsy
c *After marking at ESD*. After marking a distance 5 mm from the margin of the lesion, ESD was carried out

ous lesion can potentially be removed by biopsy, it is necessary to resect a wider area in one piece to allow detailed pathological evaluation. Such a lesion is a good candidate for ESD.

In general, endoscopically resected specimens are sliced at a thickness of 2 mm, and it is important to expose clearly the suspected site of the lesion (e.g., a biopsy scar). In this respect, ESD is more useful than EMR because the specimen obtained by ESD sustains less mechanical injury than that obtained by EMR (Refer to case 22, Early Gastric Cancer).

When a cancer might have been removed completely by biopsy, routine 2-mm slicing may leave the lesion between the incised surfaces, so the lesion is not exposed

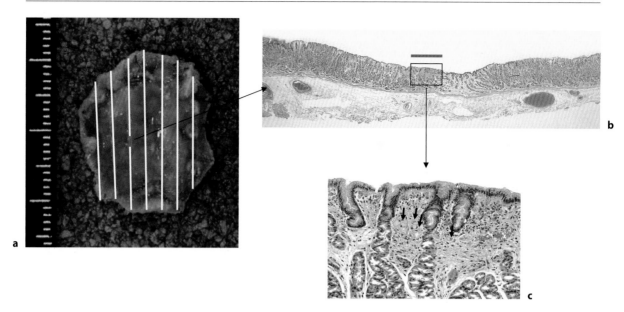

Fig. 4. a *Slicing*. Routine slicing failed to expose the lesion, so thin slicing was carried out. A "sig" lesion 2 mm in diameter was identified in only one specimen
b *With a magnifying lens*. A lesion was observed only at the surface layer of the mucosa
c *Higher magnification*. Signet-ring cells with lopsided nuclei were observed (*arrows*)

on the surface. In such cases, it is necessary to cut the specimen deeply and confirm the absence of cancerous tissue (Figs. 3, 4).

When examining the biopsied site, it is important to identify thickening of the muscularis mucosae and the presence of regenerative mucosa to confirm that the cancer has in fact disappeared after the biopsy.

The Treatment Result of Minute Cancer

A total of 483 early gastric cancers were resected endoscopically between March 2005 and August 2007 in our hospital (ESD 425, EMR 58). Among them, 77 (15.9%) were diagnosed postoperatively as minute gastric cancer. Of the 483 cases, cancer was not detected in the pathology specimen in 6 (1.2%). Minute cancer (≤5 mm in diameter) was diagnosed preoperatively in three of these six cases, and in the remaining three cases the small gastric cancer was ≤10 mm in diameter. Histological examination following biopsy revealed differentiated cancer in four cases and undifferentiated cancer in two cases. In all six cases, a 0-IIc lesion was identified macroscopically before biopsy. The average follow-up period in these six cases was 22 months, and no recurrence was observed.

Conclusion

The possibilities of complete removal of minute gastric cancer by biopsy and the follow-up strategies have been described.

References

1. Furukawa T, Kumai K, Shimada A, et al (1992) Three cases of minute gastric cancer of which cancer cells were identified in only biopsy specimen obtained from the initial endoscopic examination. Prog Dig Endosc 41:294–297
2. Nakayoshi T, Tajiri H, Matsuda K, et al (2004) Magnifying endoscopy combined with narrow band imaging system for early gastric cancer: correlation of vascular pattern with histopathology (including video). Endoscopy 36:1080–1084
3. Kato H, Sakaki N, Yamada Y, et al (1990) Changes of morphological features of minute gastric carcinomas by bite biopsy. Prog Dig Endosc 37:160–163
4. Takahashi H, Kidokoro T, Fujita R, et al (1991) Therapy of gastric cancer disappearing following biopsy (minute gastric cancer). Endosc Dig 3:341–344
5. Asaki S, Sekine H, Funada K, et al (1991) Problems associated with the diagnosis of minute gastric cancer. Endosc Dig 3:271–278
6. Machida M, Yoshida S, Tajiri H, et al (1987) Possibilities of disappearance of gastric cancer by endoscopic biopsy. Prog Dig Endosc 31:317–321
7. Tada M, Shiraishi H, Kurata S, et al (1991) A minute gastric cancer (1.5 mm) detected by strip biopsy. Endosc Dig 3:331–335
8. Gotoda T, Yamamoto H, Soetikno RM (2006) Endoscopic submucosal dissection of early gastric cancer. J Gastroenterol 41:929–942

Case Presentations: Early Gastric Cancer

Superficial Elevated Type

Case 1

63-year-old man early gastric cancer, posterior mid-body, type 0-IIa, 7-mm well-differentiated tubular adenocarcinoma (tub1).

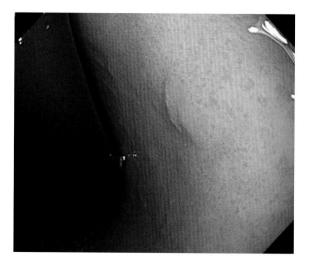

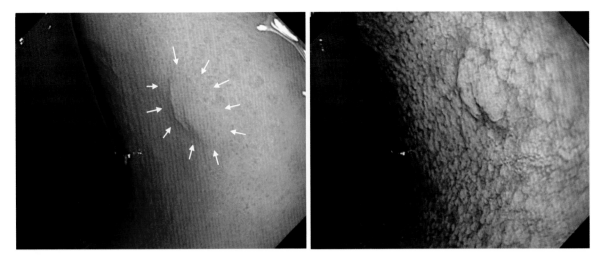

Fig. 1. Endoscopic diagnosis and findings
Routine observation: A reddish, relatively well-demarcated, flat-elevated lesion 7 mm in diameter was observed at the posterior of the mid-body of the stomach (*arrows*). The surface was slightly rough and severely reddish, similar to adjacent gastric areas. The surface was mostly flat but mildly irregular
Indigo carmine spraying: Dye spraying more clearly visualized the margin of the elevation and irregularity of the mucosal surface

Diagnostic Points:

A solitary reddish flat-elevated lesion with the background atrophic mucosa was observed.

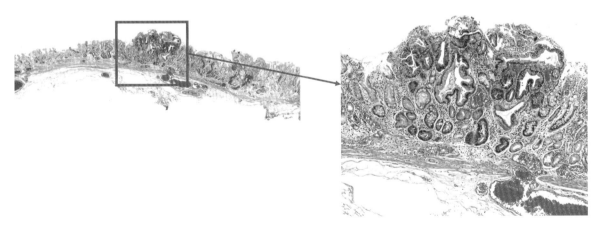

Fig. 2. *Pathological findings*
   With a magnifying lens: Cancer was recognized at almost the same area as the elevation
   Higher magnification: Higher magnification of the same region revealed well-differentiated adenocarcinoma. Cancer was confined to the mucosal layer

Case 2

61-year-old woman early gastric cancer, lesser curvature of the mid-body, type 0-IIa, 4-mm well-differentiated tubular adenocarcinoma (tub1).

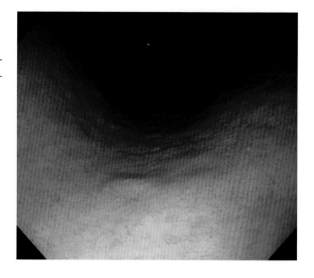

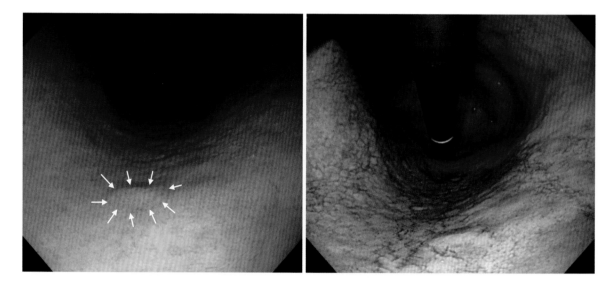

Fig. 1. Endoscopic diagnosis and findings
Routine observation: A reddish, relatively well-demarcated, flat-elevated lesion 4 mm in diameter was observed at the lesser curvature of the mid-body of the stomach (*arrows*). The mucosal surface was similar to that in adjacent gastric areas
Indigo carmine spraying: Dye spraying more clearly visualized the margin, but no marked irregularity of the surface was observed

Diagnostic Points:

A solitary reddish flat-elevated lesion was observed at the atrophic mucosa *Pathological findings*.

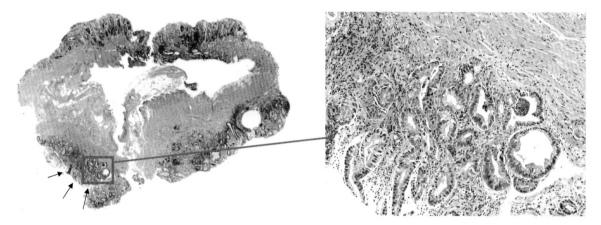

Fig. 2. *With a magnifying lens*: This specimen was resected by endoscopic mucosal resection using a cap (EMR-C). Cancer was visualized at the region indicated by the *arrows*

Higher magnification. Well-differentiated adenocarcinoma was observed in the mucosa

Superficial Flat Type

Case 3

48-year-old man early gastric cancer, greater curvature of the angle, type 0-IIb, 5-mm signet-ring cell carcinoma (sig).

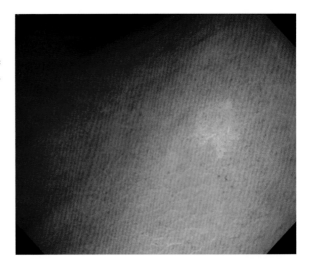

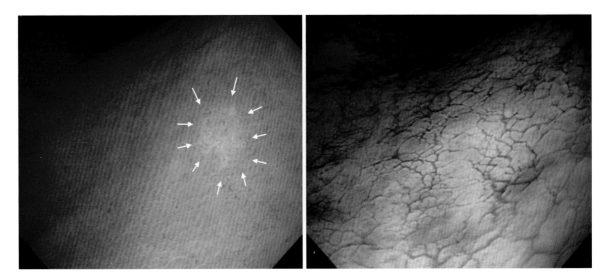

Fig. 1. Endoscopic diagnosis and findings

Routine observation: Area of discolored mucosa, 5 mm in diameter, was observed at the greater curvature of the gastric angle. The margin of the lesion was distinctly identifiable by the color change. No elevation or depression was observed in the discolored mucosa

Indigo carmine spraying: Dye spraying showed almost no difference in the lesion's surface structure compared with the adjacent mucosa, and the margin became less visible than on routine observation. This finding indicates almost no difference in lesion height compared with the adjacent mucosa

Diagnostic Points:

A solitary discolored mucosal lesion was visualized. This is a typical case with undifferentiated, superficial flat-type early gastric cancer. A minute type IIb lesion such as this exhibits little difference in surface structure compared with the adjacent normal gastric mucosa. Only color changes are seen. Because visualization of the lesion may become even more difficult with chromo-endoscopy, it is better to use first an indigo carmine solution that is more highly diluted. Should the lesion be difficult to visualize after dye spraying, the endoscopist should rinse the dye away thoroughly and reexamine the lesion.

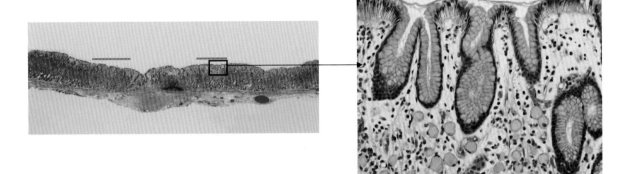

Fig. 2. *Pathohistological findings*: The lesion, completely resected by EMR in one piece, was found to be a minute signet-ring cell carcinoma. The lesion was mainly localized at the proliferative zone, and cancer was not exposed to the mucosal surface
Histology: ssg, depth M, ly0, v0, l-ce(−), v-ce(−)

Case 4

72-year-old man early gastric cancer, greater curvature of the upper body (remnant stomach), type 0-IIb, 3-mm signet-ring cell carcinoma (sig).

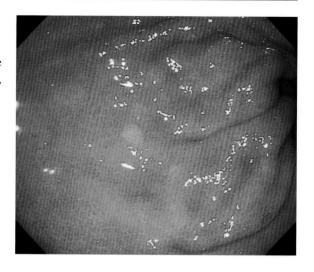

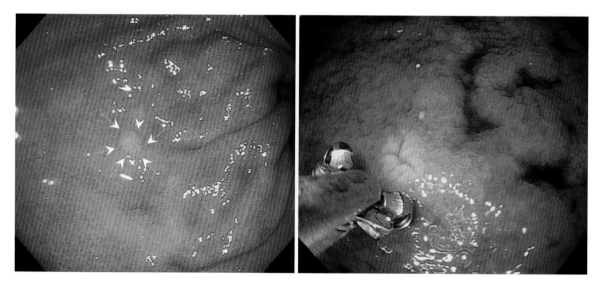

Fig. 1. Endoscopic diagnosis and findings

Routine observation: This is a remnant stomach after distal gastrectomy. A discolored lesion, 3 mm in diameter and distinctly different in color from the adjacent normal mucosa, was observed at the greater curvature of the remnant gastric body (*arrows*). The margin was well demarcated; the surface structure of the discolored lesion was relatively regular; and the color was relatively homogeneous

Indigo carmine spraying: Dye spraying revealed almost no difference in the lesion's height compared with the adjacent normal mucosa. When opened, biopsy forceps are about 5 mm wide; thus, recording an image of the lesion and forceps together is useful for measuring the lesion size objectively

Diagnostic Points:

A discolored mucosal lesion was visualized in the remnant stomach. It is known that multiple gastric cancers tend to develop synchronously or metachronously. After gastrectomy for gastric cancer, a large portion of the remaining gastric mucosa is at high risk of carcinogenesis, so close attention should be paid to the increased likelihood of metachronous carcinogenesis. For early detection of undifferentiated cancer in the remnant stomach, it is important to look for and carefully assess any color change.

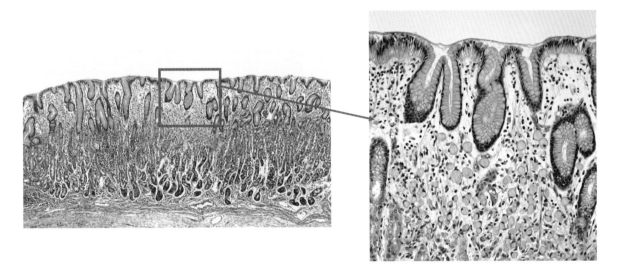

Fig. 2. *Pathohistological findings*: The lesion was completely resected in one piece by EMR
Histology: depth M, sig, ly0, v0, l-ce(−), v-ce(−)

Superficial Depressed Type

Well-Differentiated Adenocarcinoma

Case 5

80-year-old man early gastric cancer, anterior lower body, type 0-IIc, 7-mm well-differentiated adenocarcinoma.

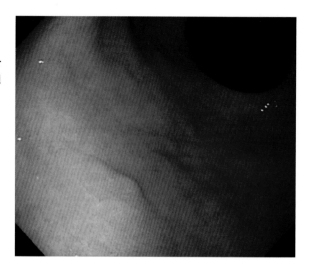

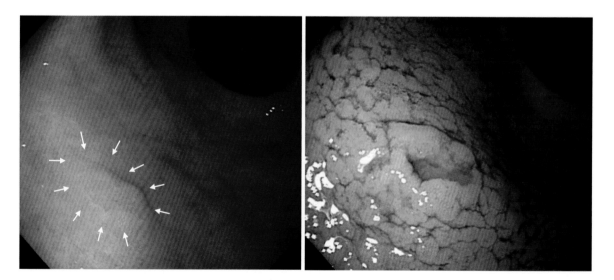

Fig. 1. Endoscopic diagnosis and findings

Routine observation: A well-demarcated depression, 7 mm in diameter, was observed at the anterior wall of the lower gastric body accompanied by surrounding elevations (*arrows*). The depression was mildly reddish, and the peripheral elevations were flat without color changes compared with the adjacent mucosa

Indigo carmine spraying: Dye spraying more clearly visualized the irregularity of the periphery of the depression and the irregularity of the depressed surface. The peripheral elevation was not steep, so a reactive elevation was suspected

Diagnostic Points:

An irregular depression was visualized accompanied by peripheral elevations.

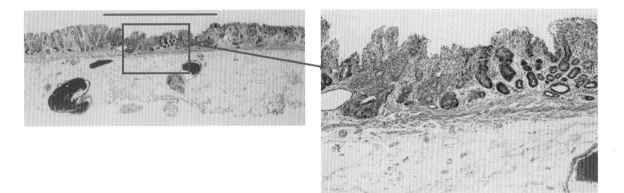

Fig. 2. *Pathohistological findings*
With a magnifying lens: This view revealed that the lesion was restricted to the depression
Higher magnification: This view showed well-differentiated adenocarcinoma limited within mucosa (depth M)

Case 6

65-year-old woman early gastric cancer, lesser curvature of the antrum, type 0-IIc, 5-mm well-differentiated tubular adenocarcinoma (tub1).

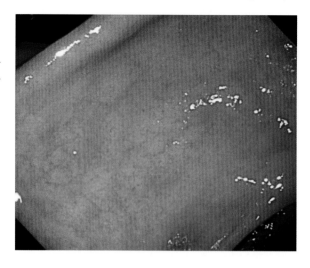

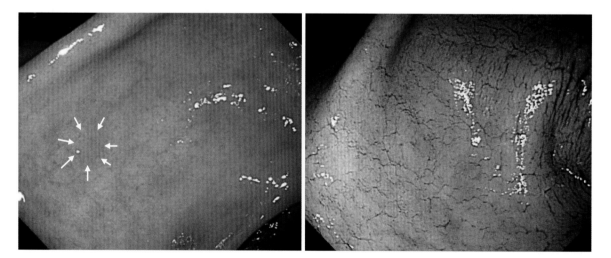

Fig. 1. Endoscopic diagnosis and findings
Routine observation: A reddish, relatively well-demarcated, flat-elevated lesion, 5 mm in diameter, was seen (*arrows*). The mucosal surface showed no marked irregularity
Indigo carmine spraying: Dye spraying more clearly visualized the margin, and the mucosal surface showed fine granular patterns, with a small depression exhibiting a slightly reddish surface at the center

Diagnostic Points:

A solitary lesion with a slightly reddish surface was visualized.

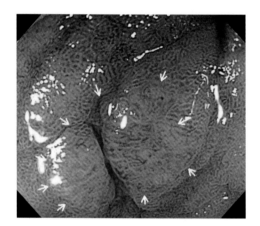

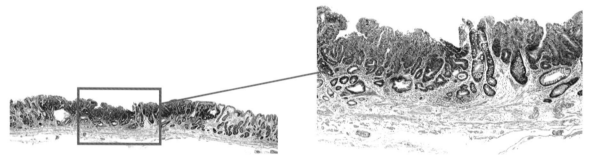

Fig. 2. *Pathological findings*
   With a magnifying lens: A slightly elevated lesion was observed. Cancer was visualized at the region corresponding to the elevation
   Higher magnification: Well-differentiated adenocarcinoma was observed in the mucosa
NBI: A well-demarcated lesion was visualized. Blood vessels were observed in the area with a cobblestone appearance

Case 7

75-year-old man early gastric cancer, lesser curvature of the mid-body, type 0-IIc, 5-mm well-differentiated tubular adenocarcinoma (tub1).

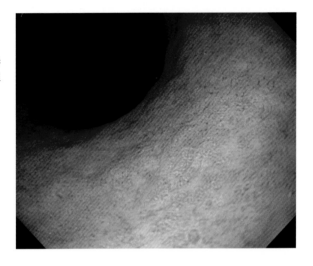

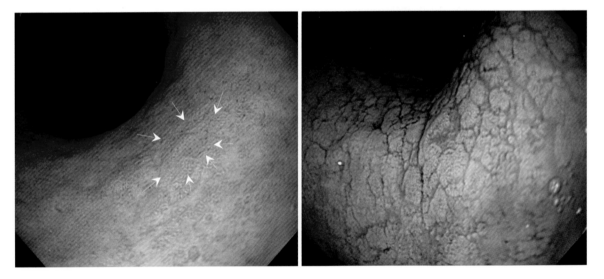

Fig. 1. Endoscopic diagnosis and findings
Routine observation: A slightly reddish, depressed lesion, about 5 mm in diameter, was observed at the lesser curvature of the gastric body (*arrows*). The depression had an unclear margin and relatively flat surface without elevation. The adjacent mucosa was slightly elevated and not firm. Thus, a reactive elevation was suspected
Indigo carmine spraying: The margin of the depression became more distinct and exhibited so-called encroachment. The surface of the depression exhibited finely granular patterns

Diagnostic Points:

A solitary, small reddish depression was visualized, with marginal encroachment. It is important not to overlook the small depression, which is distinctly different in color from the adjacent mucosa, although such small depressions are often benign erosions. Attention should be paid to their solitary presence and the patterns of the margin of the depression.

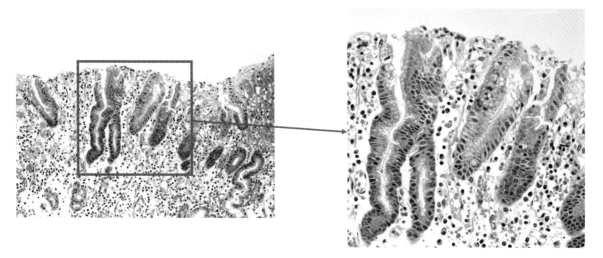

Fig. 2. *Pathohistological findings*: The lesion was completely resected in one piece by EMR
Histology: tub1, depth M, ly0, v0, l-ce(−), v-ce(−)

Case 8

69-year-old man early gastric cancer, anterior antrum, type 0-IIc, 7-mm well-differentiated adenocarcinoma (tub1).

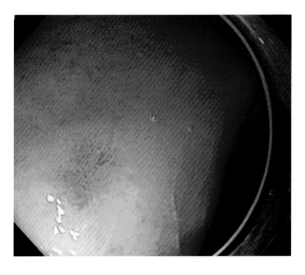

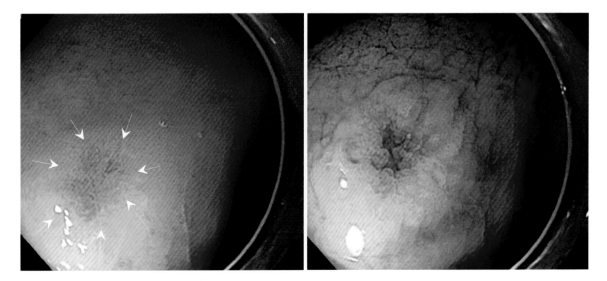

Fig. 1. Endoscopic diagnosis and findings
Routine observation: A reddish, irregular depression, 7 mm in diameter, was observed (*arrows*). The margin of the lesion was slightly unclear
Indigo carmine spraying: Dye spraying revealed encroachment at some parts of the margin of the depression. The adjacent mucosa was slightly elevated, but not steeply so, which is characteristic of a reactive elevation. Type 0-IIc well-differentiated early gastric cancer was suspected

Diagnostic Points:

The diagnosis was made possible by indigo carmine spraying, which revealed a reddish, irregular depression with encroachment.

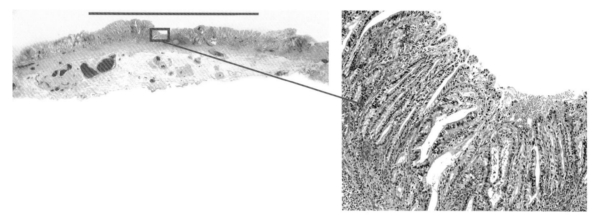

Fig. 2. *Pathohistological findings*

With a magnifying lens: This view revealed a shallow depression and infiltration of the adjacent mucosa (*red line*). Cancer was visualized not only at the reddish depression observed endoscopically but also at the adjacent reactive elevation

Higher magnification: This view revealed well-differentiated adenocarcinoma (tub1) limited within mucosa (depth M)

Case 9

68-year-old man early gastric cancer, anterior lower body, type 0-IIc, 5-mm well-differentiated adenocarcinoma (tub1).

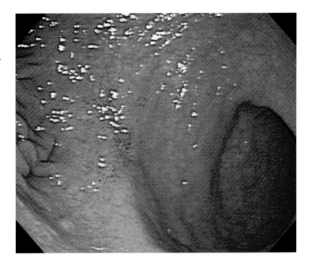

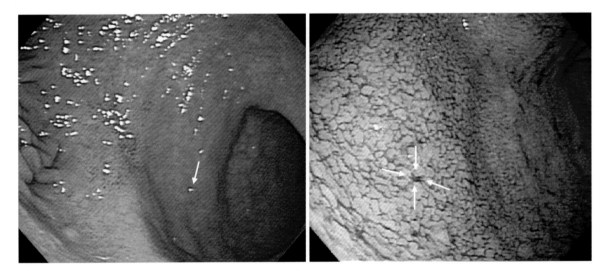

Fig. 1. Endoscopic diagnosis and findings
Routine observation: An ulcer scar (S1 stage) was observed at the anterior wall of the mid-body of the stomach accompanied by a minute depression at the anal side (*arrows*)
Indigo carmine spraying: Dye spraying more clearly visualized the depression (*arrows*) and made it easier to establish the presence of the lesion

Diagnostic Points:

Indigo carmine spraying revealed a minute reddish depression and encroachment.

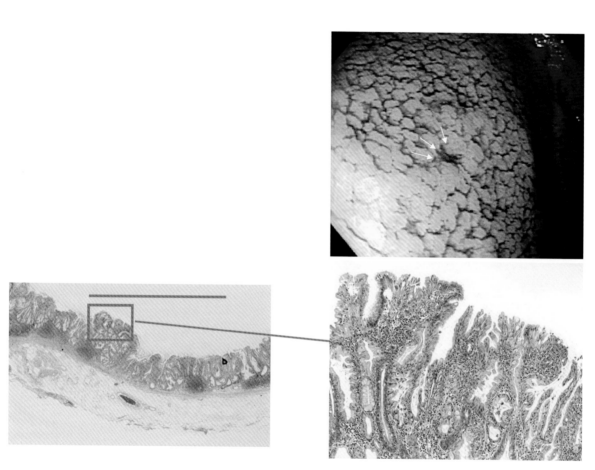

Fig. 2. *Indigo carmine spraying (close view)*: Magnified view revealed mild encroachment with extrusion from the margin of the depression (*arrows*). Type 0-IIc well-differentiated early gastric cancer was suspected
Pathohistological findings: As visualized with a magnifying lens, this view of the margin of the depression revealed that the lesion was restricted to the depression
Histology: Well-differentiated adenocarcinoma (tub1)

Case 10

69-year-old man early gastric cancer, lesser curvature of the antrum, type 0-IIc, 5-mm well-differentiated adenocarcinoma (tub1).

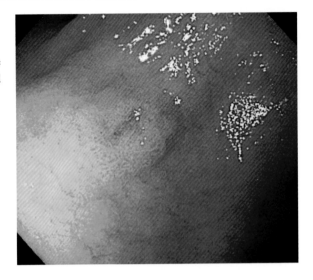

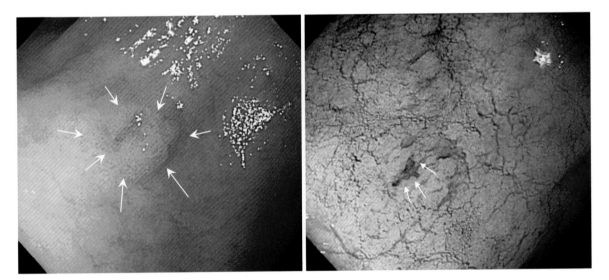

Fig. 1. Endoscopic diagnosis and findings
Routine observation: A longitudinally stretched depression, 5 mm in diameter (*arrows*), was observed. The depression's margin was unclear. A peripheral mild elevation was also observed
Indigo carmine spraying: Dye spraying revealed an irregular margin of the reddish depression, and encroachment was suspected (*arrows*). The peripheral elevation was still poorly demarcated after dye spraying

Diagnostic Points:

Recognition of a distinctly reddish depression, and the presence or absence of irregularity at the adjacent mucosa around the margin.

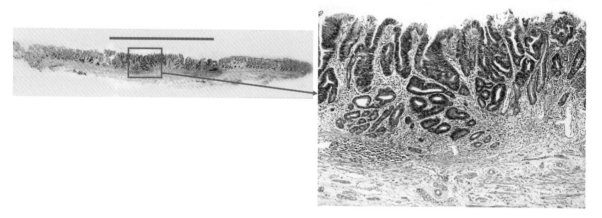

Fig. 2. Pathohistological findings

With a magnifying lens: This view revealed that the lesion was restricted to the depression (*red line*)

Higher magnification: Higher magnification of the same region revealed well-differentiated adenocarcinoma

Case 11

65-year-old woman early gastric cancer, lesser curvature of the antrum, type 0-IIc, 4-mm well-differentiated adenocarcinoma (tub1).

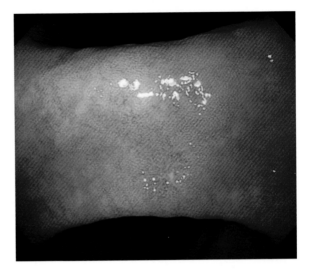

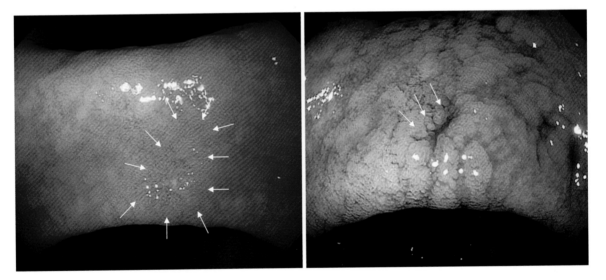

Fig. 1. Endoscopic diagnosis and findings

Routine observation: A depression, 4 mm in diameter, was observed at the lesser curvature of the gastric antrum (*arrows*). The depression was flat and partially white-coated

Indigo carmine spraying: Dye spraying more clearly visualized the margin of the lesion, including irregularity and encroachment (*arrows*). Mild redness was observed around the depression, but the boundary was indistinct, suggesting a reactive change

Diagnostic Points:

A minute white-coated depression was visualized. Diagnosis of encroachment was based on dye spraying.

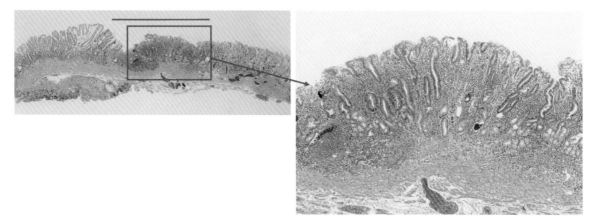

Fig. 2. *Pathohistological findings*
  With a magnifying lens: This view revealed that the cancer was restricted to the depression
  Higher magnification: This view revealed well-differentiated adenocarcinoma limited within mucosa (depth M)

Case 12

56-year-old man early gastric cancer, lesser curvature of the antrum, type 0-IIc, 5-mm well-differentiated adenocarcinoma (tub1).

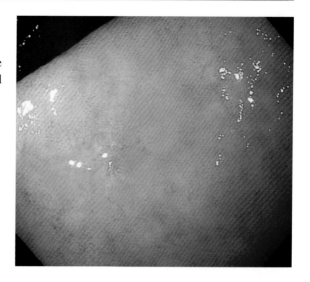

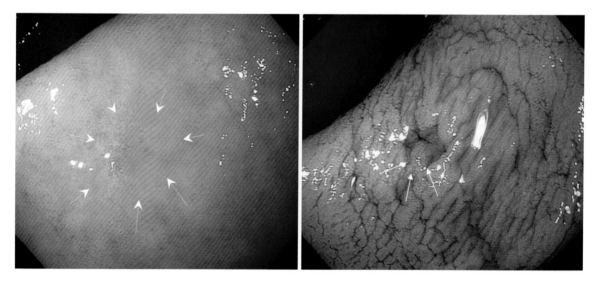

Fig. 1. Endoscopic diagnosis and findings

Routine observation: A well-demarcated, reddish depression, 5 mm in diameter, was observed at the lesser curvature of the antrum (*arrows*). The margin of the lesion was unclear

Indigo carmine spraying: Dye spraying more clearly visualized the margin of the depression, but the irregularity at the margin was mild, and encroachment was not diagnosed. Granular elevations on the depression looked like the surface of regenerative epithelium (*arrows*). The adjacent mucosa around the lesion was slightly elevated

Diagnostic Points:

A reddish depression and reactive elevations around it were visualized.

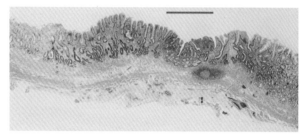
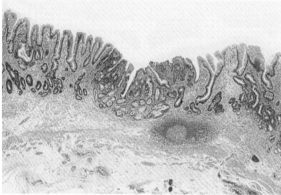

Fig. 2. *Pathohistological findings*: The lesion was slightly depressed compared with the adjacent normal mucosa, and adenocarcinoma (tub1) was recognized
Histology: adenocarcinoma (tub1), depth M, ly(–), v0, HM(–), vM(–)

Moderately Differentiated Adenocarcinoma

Case 13

61-year-old man early gastric cancer, posterior lower body, type 0-IIc, 10-mm moderately differentiated adenocarcinoma (tub2).

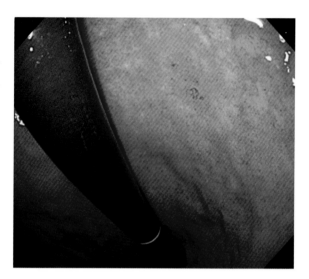

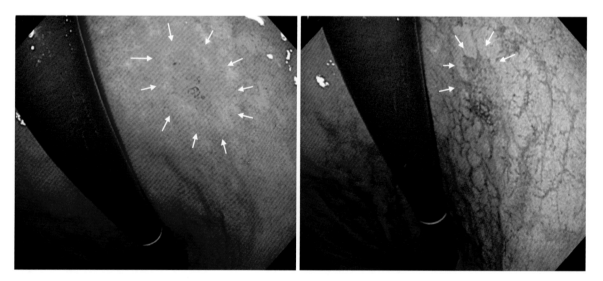

Fig. 1. Endoscopic diagnosis and findings
Routine observation: An approximately 10-mm reddish lesion that was slightly depressed compared with the adjacent mucosa was observed at the posterior wall of the lower gastric body accompanied by petechiae (*arrows*). The adjacent mucosa was atrophic
Indigo carmine spraying: Dye spraying more clearly visualized the depression. The surface of the depression was covered with reddish finely granular mucosa, and the margin was irregular with encroachment (*arrows*). These findings are suggestive of type 0-IIc early gastric cancer

Diagnostic Points:

Routine observation revealed mild redness and petechiae, suggesting the presence of a lesion. Indigo carmine spraying showed a well-demarcated depression with marginal encroachment.

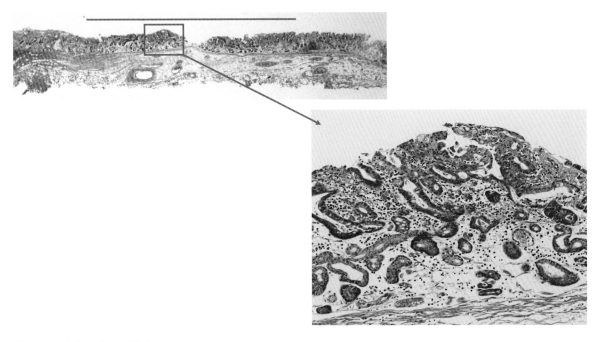

Fig. 2. *Pathohistological findings*

With a magnifying lens: This view revealed adenocarcinoma, limited with mucosa (depth M) at the depression that had been observed endoscopically

Higher magnification: This view showed marked atypia. Anastomosing-type, moderately differentiated adenocarcinoma was diagnosed

Case 14

77-year-old woman early gastric cancer, greater curvature of the antrum, type 0-IIc, 5-mm moderately differentiated adenocarcinoma (tub2).

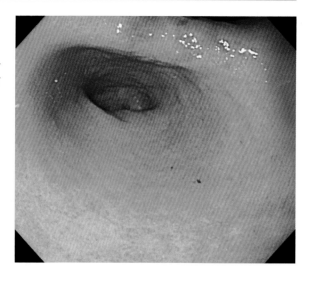

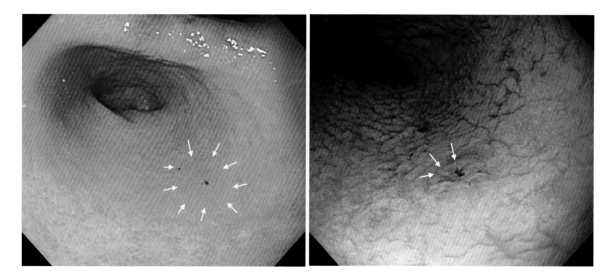

Fig. 1. Endoscopic diagnosis and findings

Routine observation: A small erosion, 5 mm in diameter, with blood clot was observed in the greater curvature of the antrum (*arrows*). These erosions were not seen in the adjacent mucosa

Indigo carmine spraying: Dye spraying more clearly visualized the depression (*arrows*). The margin of the depression was irregular, and encroachment was suspected. Mild elevations were observed in the periphery, but the boundary was unclear

Diagnostic Points:

Routine observation revealed a small amount of blood clot. Indigo carmine spraying showed an irregular margin, which suggested encroachment.

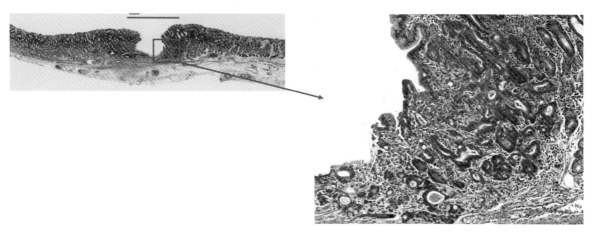

Fig. 2. *Pathohistological findings*: The lesion, restricted to the depression, was moderately differentiated adenocarcinoma that had formed small cancer glands with irregular branching and convergence

Case 15

69-year-old man early gastric cancer, lesser curvature of the antrum, type 0-IIc, 5-mm moderately differentiated adenocarcinoma (tub2).

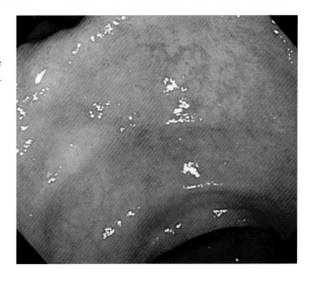

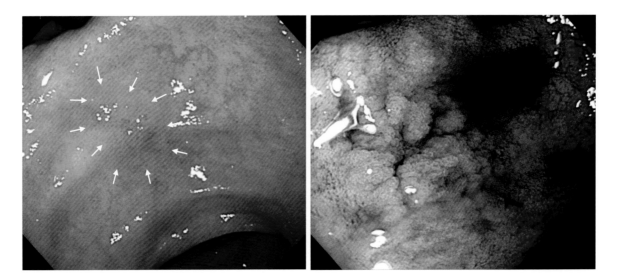

Fig. 1. Endoscopic diagnosis and findings
Routine observation: A lesion with redness, 5 mm in diameter and lacking visible blood vessels in the adjacent atrophic mucosa, was observed at the lesser curvature of the antrum (*arrows*)
Indigo carmine spraying: Dye spraying revealed a gutter-like depression at the center of the site, without visible blood vessels. The depression had an irregular margin, and the peripheral mucosa was slightly elevated, which seemed to be a reactive change

Diagnostic Points:

Atrophic mucosa and disappearance of visible blood vessels were observed during routine observation. A gutter-like depression with an irregular margin was revealed by dye spraying.

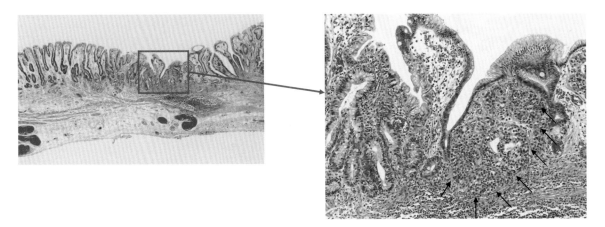

Fig. 2. *Pathohistological findings*

With a magnifying lens: This view revealed that the lesion was slightly depressed compared with the adjacent mucosa. The cancerous lesion was restricted to the depression

Higher magnification: This view showed swollen nuclei of the cancer cells, and columnar or cubic cells with perturbed polarity formed cancer with small to medium-sized glands. For the most part, gland formation was unclear, and a solid-type poorly differentiated adenocarcinoma with dense growth of atypical cells was diagnosed (*arrows*)

Case 16

66-year-old woman early gastric cancer, lesser curvature of the antrum, type 0-IIc, 3-mm moderately differentiated adenocarcinoma (tub2).

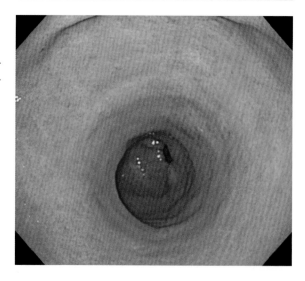

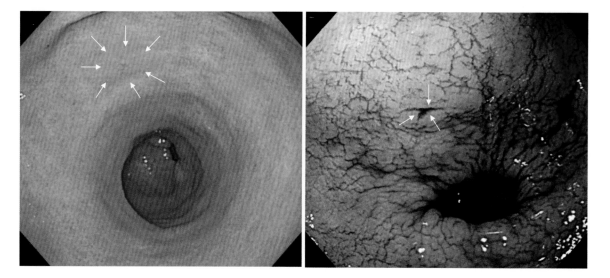

Fig. 1. Endoscopic diagnosis and findings

Routine observation: A pale pink mucosal lesion was observed at the lesser curvature of the antrum (*arrows*), with a mildly depressed whitish center

Indigo carmine spraying: Dye spraying revealed that redness was present on a diamond-shaped, mildly elevated area that was longer transversely and had a well-demarcated depression at the center (*arrows*). This depression gave the impression of irregularity upon routine observation. It was 3 mm in size, like a gutter, with fine lines stretching from the center (like spider legs). The depression was relatively wide at the center. No granular change or elevation was observed in the depression

Diagnostic Points:

Macroscopically, the lesion was seen as mucosa with redness. The depression observed using dye spraying exhibited spikes (or a star with several peaks). The depression showed encroachment in some parts. In general, reddish depressions with irregularity are often differentiated adenocarcinoma.

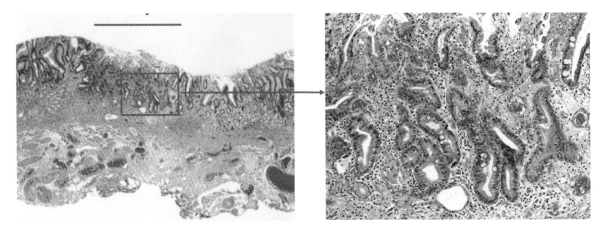

Fig. 2. *Pathohistological findings*: The lesion had characteristics of cancer, such as heterogeneity in nuclear size and increased chromatin density. The tubular structure was recognized, but their irregularity was marked. Moderately differentiated adenocarcinoma (tub2) was diagnosed. It seemed that vascular dilatation in the mucosa was present
Histology: depth M, tub2, ly0, v0, v-ce(−), l-ce(−)

Signet-Ring Cell Carcinoma

Case 17

73-year-old woman early gastric cancer, greater curvature of the antrum, type 0-IIc, 10-mm signet-ring
cell carcinoma (sig).

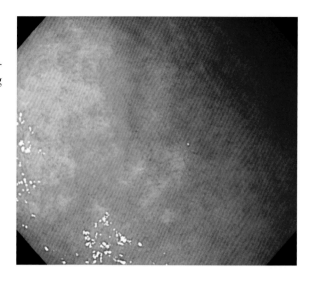

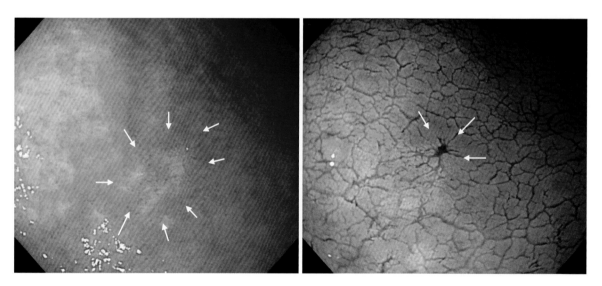

Fig. 1. Endoscopic diagnosis and findings
Routine observation: Background mucosa was atrophic, so whitish and reddish mucosae were alternately aligned. A discolored
lesion, 10 mm in diameter, was observed at the greater curvature of the antrum (*arrows*). The discolored lesion exhibited an irregular
shape (like a comet with a tail), and the margin was clear. It seemed that there was a small depression at the anal side, corresponding to the core of the comet
Indigo carmine spraying: Dye spraying revealed an even, unclear margin of discoloration but a clear margin of the depression. A
small, irregular depression corresponding to the comet's core became particularly evident (*arrows*). There was no encroachment.
Several gutter-like depressions extended to the proximal side like a crack and corresponded to the region with discoloration seen
macroscopically. The lesion was diagnosed macroscopically as type 0-IIc with invasion into the mucosa (depth M) and histologically as poorly differentiated adenocarcinoma (based on the discoloration)

Diagnostic Points:

An asymmetrical lesion with discolored mucosa and a depression at the center of the lesion was visualized. The margin of the depression was clear, but the lesion itself became unclear when examined after dye spraying.

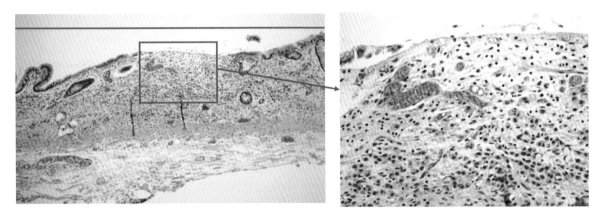

Fig. 2. *Pathohistological findings*: Tubular structure was not recognized, and signet-ring cells were observed. Few blood vessels were seen
Histology: depth M, por2, sig, ly0, v0, L-ce(−), v-ce(−)

Case 18

68-year-old man early gastric cancer, greater curvature of the mid-body, type 0-IIc, 8-mm signet-ring cell carcinoma (sig).

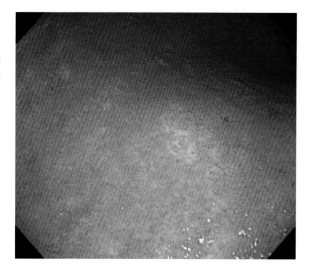

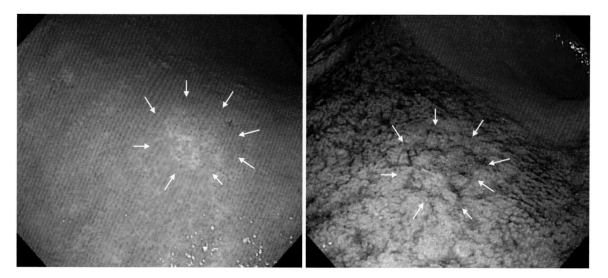

Fig. 1. Endoscopic diagnosis and findings

Routine observation: The background mucosa was widely atrophic, and it seemed that a large amount of white mucus was attached to the mucosa, possibly due to the presence of *Helicobacter pylori*. A discolored region, 5–6 mm in diameter and with an unclear margin, was evident at the greater curvature of the angle (*arrows*). The center of the rugby ball-shaped mild discoloration was more whitish, and blood vessels were more clearly observed at the anal side. The area looked slightly depressed compared with the adjacent mucosa

Indigo carmine spraying: Because of the presence of mucus, the boundary of the discoloration became more unclear. However, the mucosa at the center was clearly visualized as an irregular depression (*arrows*). A gap in height and discoloration were evident, and the margin was irregular but not as clear as in case 19 (see later). Collectively, the lesion was diagnosed as type 0-IIc, limited within mucosa (depth M) seen macroscopically. It was a depressed lesion with discoloration, and undifferentiated histology was suspected

Diagnostic Points:

Discolored mucosa was visualized.

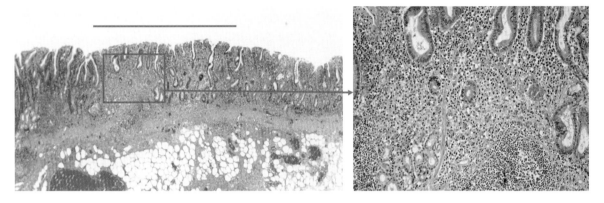

Figs. 2. *Pathohistological findings*: A normal glandular structure with low density was observed, and signet-ring cells were identified in the lesion. Compared with adjacent mucosa, the vascular density was low, and therefore the lesion appeared discolored endoscopically
Histology: depth M, sig, ly0, v0, L-ce(−), v-ce(−)

Case 19

33-year-old woman early gastric cancer, greater curvature of the angle, type 0-IIc, 8-mm signet-ring cell
carcinoma (sig).

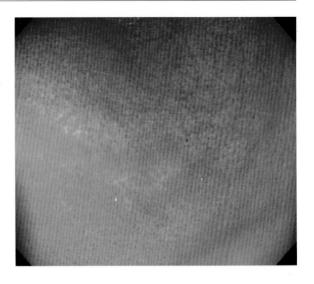

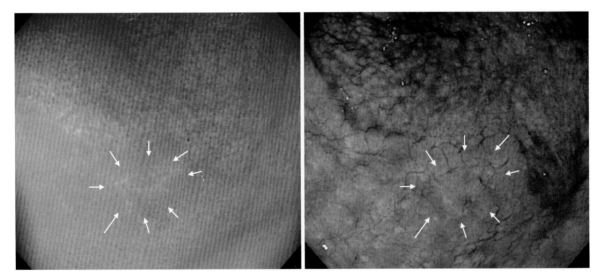

Fig. 1. Endoscopic diagnosis and findings
Routine observation: The background mucosa showed closed-type atrophy; and goosebump-like lymphoid follicle hyperplasia was
scattered in the gastric body. The atrophy boundary was visualized at the greater curvature of the gastric angle, and a mesh-like
discolored region, about 8 × 4 mm in diameter and with an unclear margin, was evident in the nonatrophic mucosa (*arrows*). It
seemed that the distal area to the discoloration was slightly depressed
Indigo carmine spraying: Dye spraying rendered the margin of the discolored area ambiguous, but there was a depression at the
center (*arrows*). The distal side of the depression was relatively wider, and other parts were visualized as a twisted gutter-like
depression that had no elevation or redness at the center. There was no ulcer scar. Collectively, the macroscopic diagnosis was
type 0-IIc, depth M. The lesion was a discolored depression, and undifferentiated histology was suspected

Diagnostic Points:

Discoloration in the nonatrophic mucosa was visualized. A well-demarcated depression was observed at the center of the lesion. The periphery of the depression was gutter-like and twisted.

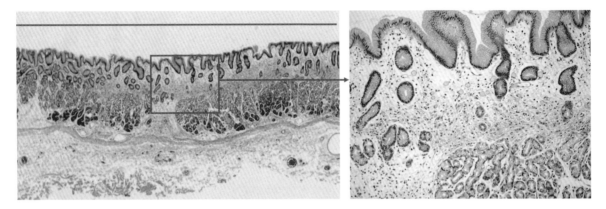

Fig. 2. *Pathohistological findings*: A tubular structure was relatively preserved, but signet-ring cells were observed. It seems that the area with low vascular density was visualized as discoloration
Histology: depth M, sig, ly0, v0, v-ce(–), l-ce(–)

Case 20

58-year-old woman early gastric cancer, posterior mid-body, type 0-IIc, 2-mm signet-ring cell carcinoma (sig).

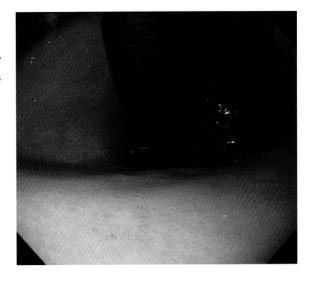

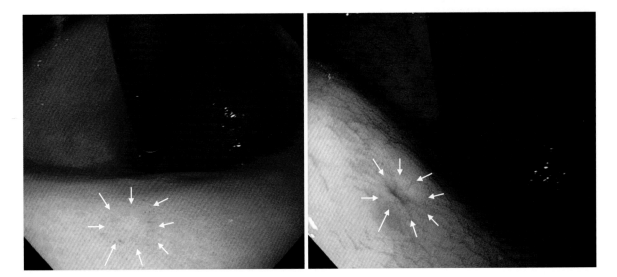

Fig. 1. Endoscopic diagnosis and findings

Routine observation: The background mucosa was mildly atrophic and slightly reddish. A minute, whitish mucosal area was observed at the posterior wall of the mid-body of the stomach (*arrows*). The area was clearly distinguished from the adjacent mucosa because of the small reddish spots around it. There was no elevation

Indigo carmine spraying: Dye spraying revealed a small, almost square depression, 3 mm in diameter, with a clear margin (*arrows*). The depression was not steep but was well demarcated. There was no irregularity at the margin, and no elevation was present on the depression. Macroscopic diagnosis was type 0-IIc, depth M. Based on the findings of discoloration and a relatively distinct difference in height, poorly differentiated adenocarcinoma was suspected

Diagnostic Points:

A distinct, discolored depression was present in the mildly atrophic mucosa. For detection of an extremely small lesion such as this, it is important to examine the lesion under optimal conditions (i.e., at a close distance and setting the monitor's exposure switch at "peak").

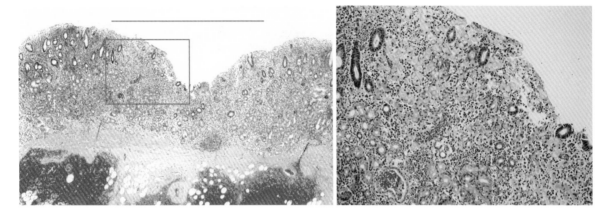

Fig. 2. *Pathohistological findings*: The lesion had a normal glandular structure of low density, and some signet-ring cells were observed. Vascular density was low. Infiltration of small, spherical inflammatory cells was observed at the periphery
Histology: depth M, sig, 2 mm, ly0, v0, v-ce(−), l-ce(−)

Case 21

59-year-old woman early gastric cancer, lesser curvature of the lower body, type 0-IIc, 5-mm signet-ring
cell carcinoma (sig).

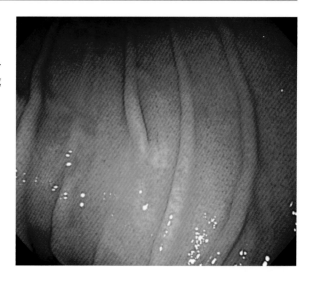

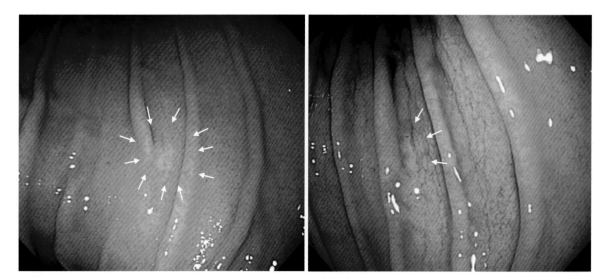

Fig. 1. Endoscopic diagnosis and findings
Routine observation: Compared with the adjacent mucosa, a 5-mm slightly discolored area was observed at the lesser curvature
of the lower body (*arrows*). Regular arrangement of collecting venules (RAC) was recognized in the adjacent mucosa, which
indicated no mucosal atrophy
Indigo carmine spraying: Dye spraying revealed neither a distinct depression at the boundary of the discolored area nor encroachment at the margin. The discolored region showed findings similar to those in the adjacent gastric areas (*arrows*). Dye spraying
rendered the color change less distinct when compared with the adjacent mucosa

Diagnostic Points:

A minute discolored area with disappearing RAC was seen in the nonatrophic mucosa by routine observation. Color changes were less distinct after indigo carmine spraying.

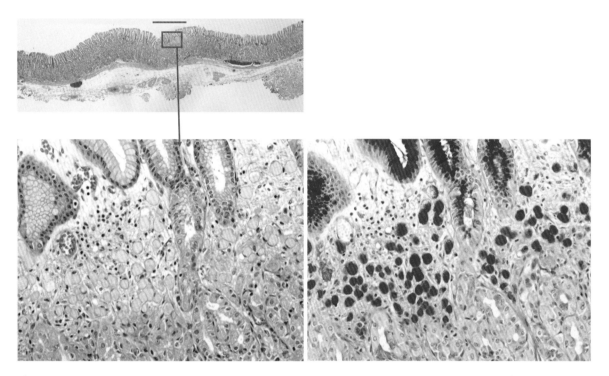

Fig. 2. *Pathohistological findings*
With a magnifying lens: This view showed that the mucosa of the lesion and the adjacent mucosa were of comparable thickness, and nonatrophic gastric fundic glands were observed
Higher magnification: This view showed signet-ring cells at the proliferative zone of the mucosa. The mucus of the cancer cells were positive for PAS staining

Scratch Cancer

Case 22

66-year-old woman early gastric cancer, posterior angle, type 0-IIc, 5-mm well-differentiated tubular adenocarcinoma (tub1).

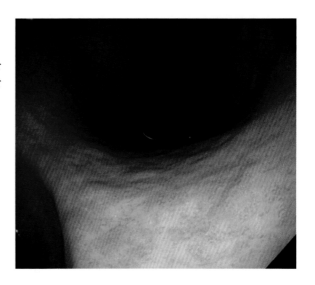

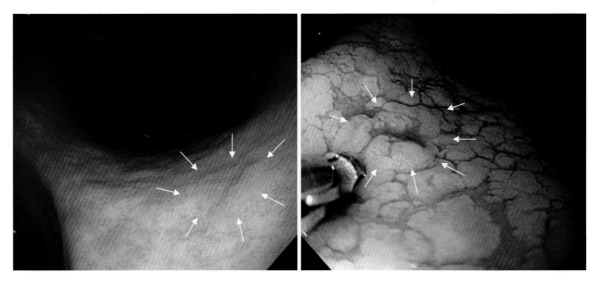

Fig. 1. Endoscopic diagnosis and findings
Routine observation: A reddish depressed lesion with peripheral mild elevation was observed in the atrophic mucosa at the posterior wall of the gastric angle (*arrows*)
Indigo carmine spraying: Encroachment was observed at the periphery of the depression accompanied by mild redness at the periphery (*arrows*). Using the biopsy forceps for comparison, the lesion was estimated to be 5 mm in diameter. Type 0-IIc early gastric cancer was suspected

Diagnostic Points:

A slightly reddish depression was seen by routine observation, with encroachment revealed by indigo carmine spraying.

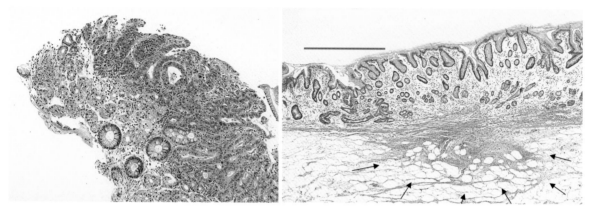

Fig. 2. *Pathohistological findings*

Biopsy specimen: Glandular density was high, and glandular atypia was recognized. Nuclei of the glands with atypia were swollen, and a multilayered structure was evident. These findings are characteristic of well-differentiated adenocarcinoma

ESD specimen: Well-differentiated adenocarcinoma was observed in only one specimen, and an intramucosal cancer, 2 mm in diameter, was present. Thickening of the muscularis mucosae close to the lesion (possibly a change due to the biopsy) was observed (*arrows*). It is probable that part of the lesion was removed by biopsy, so the lesion is now smaller

Case 1

46-year-old man 6-mm gastric carcinoid in the posterior wall of the mid-body.

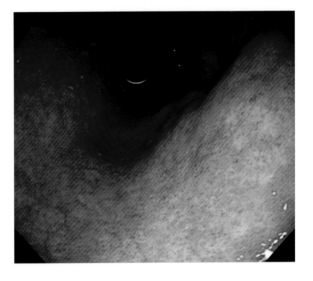

 Fujita, Takahashi (Eds.), *Gastrointestinal Cancer Atlas for Endoscopic Therapy*, DOI: 10.1007/978-4-431-88166-7_7
© Springer

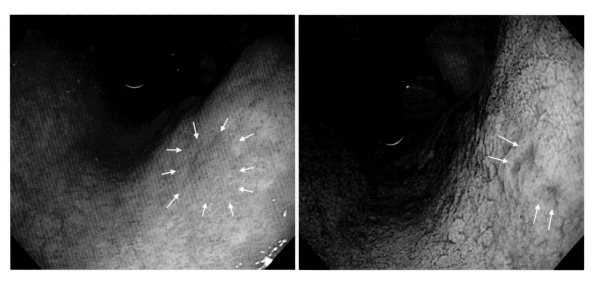

Fig. 1. Endoscopic diagnosis and findings
Routine observation: A slightly reddish, ill-demarcated, flat-elevated lesion 6 mm in diameter was observed on the atrophic mucosa at the posterior wall of the lesser curvature of the mid-body (*arrows*). The surface was irregular
Indigo carmine spraying: Dye spraying rendered the elevation margin slightly clearer, and depressions were observed at two sites on the elevated area (*arrows*). No distinct encroachment was observed at the depression

Diagnostic Points:

A typical carcinoid exhibits elevation without a sharp rise, and its surface is comparable to that of the adjacent mucosa, a common finding for submucosal tumors. It is also characterized by a yellowish color and dilated capillaries visible on the surface. No typical findings for carcinoid were observed in this case.

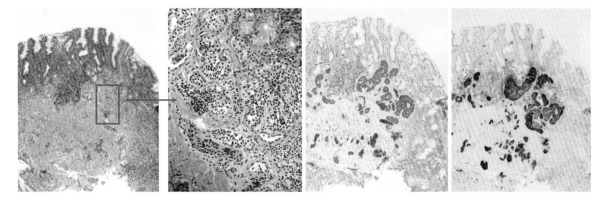

Fig. 2. *Pathohistological findings*: Heterogeneous small cells with weakly eosinophilic cytoplasm and oval or spherical nuclei with scanty polymorphism were arranged in strands at the deep part of the mucosa, exhibiting an alveolar shape. No nuclear fission was observed
Immunohistochemistry: positive staining for chromogranin A (*2nd from right*), synaptophysin (*right*), and neural cell adhesion molecule (NCAM)

Case 1

70-year-old man 3-mm carcinoid in the anterior aspect of the duodenal bulb.

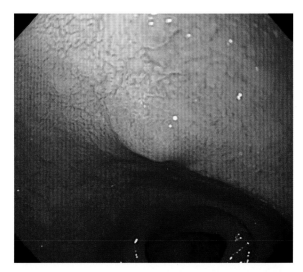

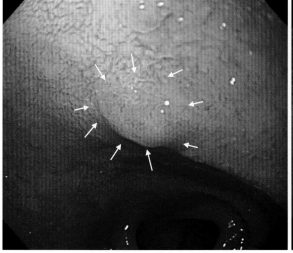

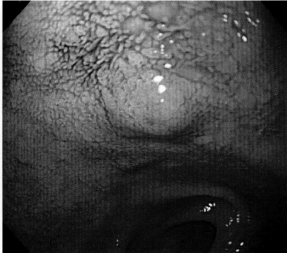

Fig. 1. Endoscopic diagnosis and findings

Routine observation: A gradually elevated lesion 3 mm in size (*arrows*) was observed at the lesser curvature of the duodenal bulb. The mucosa at the margin was villous and comparable to the adjacent mucosa, but the center was mildly reddish and villous structure was obscure

Indigo carmine spraying: Indigo carmine spraying more clearly visualized the elevation. A slightly reddish depression was observed on the top

Fujita, Takahashi (Eds.), *Gastrointestinal Cancer Atlas for Endoscopic Therapy*, DOI: 10.1007/978-4-431-88166-7_8
© Springer

Diagnostic Points:

The lesion was localized in the proximity of the pyloric ring at the anterior wall of the duodenal bulb. This site may be overlooked unless an endoscope is first inserted into the duodenal bulb and then pulled until the area nearest the pyloric ring can be visualized. Large carcinoids may have a central depression. In this case, the findings at the center suggested the process of creating a depression was under way.

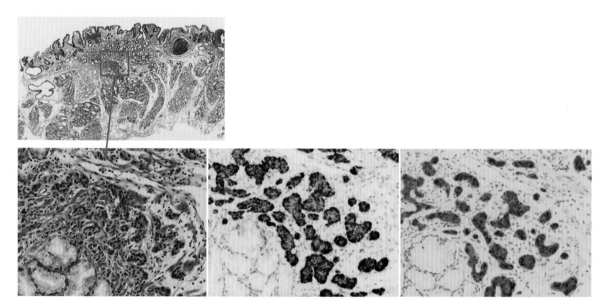

Fig. 2. Pathohistological findings
The volume of the carcinoid tumor have been decreased by the biopsy. Heterogeneous small cells with weakly eosinophilic cytoplasm and oval or spherical nuclei with scanty polymorphism were arrayed in strands at the deep part of the mucosa. No nuclear fission was observed. Immunohistochemistry: positive staining for chromogranin A (*bottom middle*), synaptophysin (*bottom right*)

Case 2

58-year-old woman 4-mm carcinoid in the anterior aspect of the duodenal bulb.

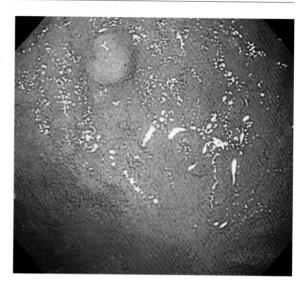

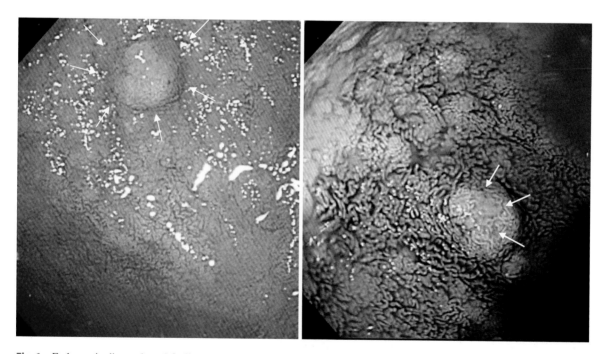

Fig. 1. Endoscopic diagnosis and findings

Routine observation: A lesion with gradual elevation, 4 mm in diameter, was visualized at the anterior wall of the duodenal bulb (*arrows*)

Indigo carmine spraying: Dye spraying revealed villi at the elevated margin, as in the adjacent mucosa; but a slightly reddish depression was observed on the top, where the villi had become obscure (*arrows*)

Diagnostic Points:

This elevated lesion showed a gradual rise. A depression was present on the top.

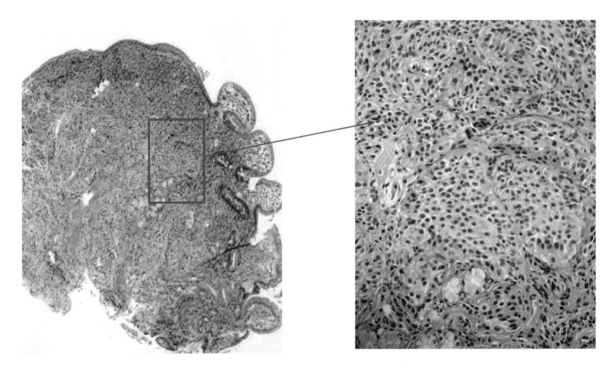

Fig. 2. *Pathohistological findings*: Homogeneous small cells with weakly eosinophilic cytoplasm and oval or spherical nuclei with scanty polymorphism were arranged in strands at the middle part of the mucosa, exhibiting an alveolar shape. Carcinoid was not observed after several biopsy sessions, and it was suspected that the lesion had been completely removed by biopsy

Case 3

75-year-old man early duodenal cancer, major papilla, type 0-IIa, 8-mm well-differentiated adenocarcinoma (tub1).

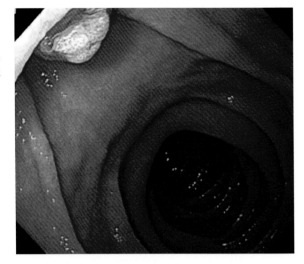

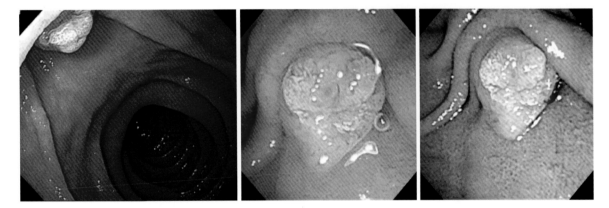

Fig. 1. Endoscopic diagnosis and findings

Routine observation: The lesion was viewed tangentially by routine endoscopic observation, but the entire papilla could not be observed from this angle, although part of the swollen papilla with a whitish granular pattern was visualized. Biopsy from this site led to the diagnosis of well-differentiated adenocarcinoma

Side-viewing endoscopy: For further scrutiny, reexamination with a side-viewing endoscope allowed a view of the papilla from the front and a complete image of the tumor. The swollen tumor was localized at the orifice, and whitish and slightly reddish areas were mixed. The surface of the mucosa revealed granules of heterogeneous size

Indigo carmine spraying: Dye spraying revealed a lesion distinctly separated from the normal structure and located at the orifice on the elevation

Diagnostic Points:

Observation of the duodenal papilla with a front-viewing endoscope (called a pan-endoscope) is often difficult because the papilla is viewed tangentially. However, swelling of the papilla and a marked color change are sufficiently recognizable. For a screening examination of the upper gastrointestinal tract with a panendoscope, it is important to pay close attention to the duodenum; and when findings of swelling of the papilla and mild redness are observed, biopsy should be performed.

A side-viewing endoscope is ideally suited for viewing the lesion from the front. Tumors arising from the duodenal papilla include adenoma, cancer, and neuroendocrine tumors.

As in this case, swelling of the papilla at the orifice along with granular changes on the mucosal surface often indicate cancer arising from the common duct and the biliary and pancreatic ducts at the papilla. Adenomas, in contrast, often arise not from the orifice but from the adjacent duodenal mucosa. Hence, evaluation of the tumor type based on the location of the lesion is key to the diagnosis.

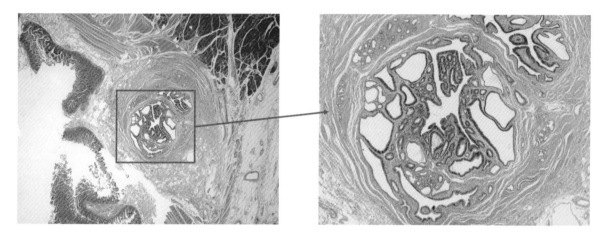

Fig. 2. *Pathohistological findings*: Endoscopic resection was attempted but resulted in incomplete resection; therefore, pancreatoduodenectomy was performed. Differentiated adenocarcinoma derived from the duodenal papilla and common duct was diagnosed

Histology: localization of PatAc, well-differentiated adenocarcinoma (tub1), ly0, v0, pn0, depth M, panc0, du0, bm0, dm0, pm0, em0

Part **IV**
Colon

Endoscopic Diagnosis of Small and Minute Colorectal Cancers

Masahiro Igarashi

Introduction

Clearly, colorectal cancer lesions do not suddenly appear at a size of 10–20 mm in diameter. Instead, they arise from minute cancers (≤5 mm) that grow into small cancers (>5 to 10 mm). Clinically, the probability of detecting a minute cancer is low (1). Small lesions such as adenomas and hyperplastic polyps account for an overwhelmingly large proportion of those detected by endoscopy (2). Hence, it is difficult to find such cancers with ordinary observation.

Endoscopic Diagnosis

To detect minute colorectal cancer, ideally there is no residue in the bowel and no mucus attached to the mucosa. Bowel preparation is essential for the detection of minute cancer. Also important is the use of a high-resolution endoscopic system for the examination (3). Movement of the bowel should be limited and the mucosa easily extended or shrunk by insufflation and desufflation of air. Therefore, an anticholinergic agent is useful for premedication.

Key Points for Observation

Points that are key to successful detection of small and minute colorectal lesions are as follows.

- Be observant and aware of the potential presence of superficial-type tumors. It is not possible to detect depressed-type and superficial-type lesions unless the endoscopist is fully aware of their potential presence and takes great care to be observant during the examination.
- Observe by controlling the air volume. It is important to focus on the irregularity of the folds and color changes during the observation by expanding and deflating the bowel. At the same time, the endoscopist can enhance the examination views by rinsing the mucosa when necessary to keep the lumen clean.

Fujita, Takahashi (Eds.), *Gastrointestinal Cancer Atlas for Endoscopic Therapy*, DOI: 10.1007/978-4-431-88166-7_9
© Springer

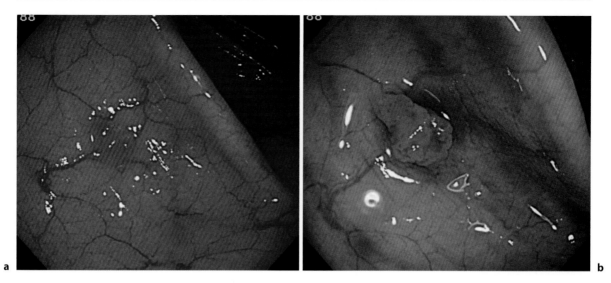

Fig. 1. Endoscopic view of colorectal lesion: redness (**a**) and surface after dye spraying (**b**)

- Focus on color changes. Minute superficial-type and depressed-type tumors are observed as redness (Fig. 1a). It is important to spray indigo carmine to clarify the surface structure and texture of the lesion (Fig. 1b).
- Pay attention to the morphological changes of the margins of the folds. Extension of the lesion onto the fold may become a key to detection.
- Be cautious about bleeding and white patches. When a lesion is cancerous, it is likely to bleed, which may be a key sign that facilitates detection. Sometimes white patches exist around the lesion.

With regard to macroscopic morphology, cancer can be categorized into the protruded type and the superficial/depressed type. It has been recognized that the probability of containing cancer cells is low in the protruded type but high in the superficial type (4, 5). In terms of the depth of invasion, cancer confined to the mucosal layer (M) is often observed, whereas cancer—with invasion to the submucosal layer (SM), ≤5 mm—is rarely found (6, 7). Accordingly, because of the low probability of protruded-type minute polyps containing cancer cells, it is generally considered unnecessary to resect them endoscopically (8). However, because even minute lesions (≤5 mm) may contain cancer cells, indications for endoscopic resection should be determined after ruling out adenomas and hyperplastic polyps that do not require treatment. Keys to differentiation are discussed below.

Differentiating Tumors from Nontumors

Endoscopic findings were compared between colorectal tumors and hyperplastic polyps (Fig. 2). In terms of color, 82% of tumors exhibited redness, whereas 62% of hyperplastic polyps were whitish or a color comparable to that of the adjacent mucosa (Table 1). Morphologically, tumors may exhibit pedunculated, semipedunculated, and sessile forms, whereas most hyperplastic polyps are sessile; differentia-

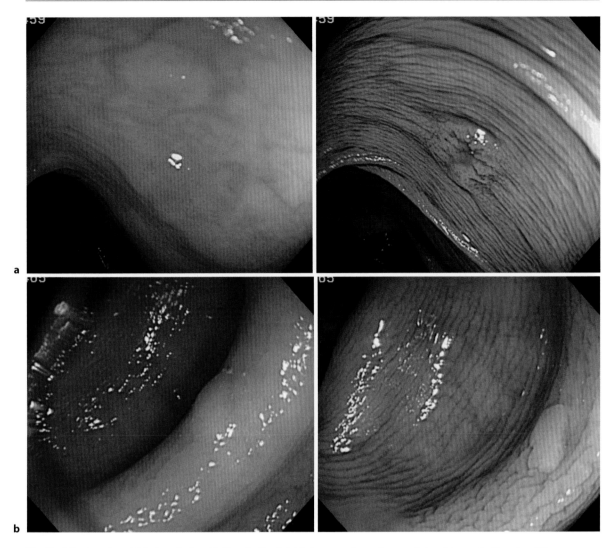

Fig. 2. Minute colorectal lesions before (*left*) and after (*right*) dye spraying: adenoma (**a**) and hyperplastic polyp (**b**)

Table 1. Correlation between surface color and histology of colorectal lesions

Histological diagnosis	Redness	Same color as mucosa	Pale	Total
Adenoma (no.)	170	20	17	207
Hyperplastic polyp (no.)	35	10	46	91

tion by routine comprehensive endoscopic observation was possible in more than 90% (Table 2). Furthermore, addition of magnifying observation with narrow band imaging (NBI) increases the diagnostic accuracy. Magnifying endoscopy shows the type II pit pattern in hyperplastic polyps and the type III–V pit patterns in tumors, which is useful for the differential diagnosis (9). When NBI and magnifying endoscopy are combined, hyperplastic polyps can be differentiated based on the characteristic of scanty vascular components (10).

Table 2. Diagnostic differentiation of colorectal adenoma from hyperplastic polyp by endoscopy or histology

Endoscopic diagnosis	Histological diagnosis (no.)		Accuracy (%)
	Adenoma	Hyperplastic polyp	
Adenoma	190	17	92
Hyperplastic polyp	6	85	93

Table 3. Correlation between endoscopic findings and macroscopic type for minute (≤5 mm diameter) colorectal cancers

Macroscopic type	Depressed area	Friable	Uneven mucosa
Protruded (n = 18)	0	3 (17%)	1 (6%)
Superficial (n = 12)	6 (50%)	2 (17%)	1 (8%)

Differentiating Cancer from Adenoma

Surface irregularity, depression, heterogeneity, and bleeding tendency are endoscopic findings suggestive of M cancers, whereas findings suggestive of SM cancers include fullness, marked depression, surface irregularity, amorphous changes, protrusion in the depression, an elevated pedestal, and fold convergence (11). Because most protruded-type minute cancers (≤5 mm) are m cancers, these findings are difficult to observe. However, even minute lesions may exhibit findings suggestive of cancer, so it is necessary always to pay close attention during the endoscopic evaluation.

On the other hand, superficial-type minute cancers often show areas of depression (Table 3). Because these cancers are often observed as red patches during routine endoscopic examinations, attention should be paid to such lesions. When they are detected, it is important to focus on the depression after spraying indigo carmine (0.2% v/v). When a depressed surface with a curve is observed, cancer should be suspected and endoscopic mucosal resection (EMR) performed for a histological diagnosis.

Small cancers (>5 to 10 mm) show more distinct endoscopic findings, as previously mentioned (Fig. 3), so the diagnosis becomes relatively easy.

Conclusion

The steps necessary for successful diagnosis of minute and small colorectal cancers are summarized in Fig. 4. During observation, the endoscopist should always rinse off any residue and mucus. With the focus on redness and morphological changes of the folds, dye spraying should be carried out when a tumor is suspected. Detected lesions then must be evaluated as tumors or nontumors, and magnifying endoscopy and NBI observation should be added. When a tumor is diagnosed and cancer is suspected, the tumor should be completely excised by EMR and examined histologically.

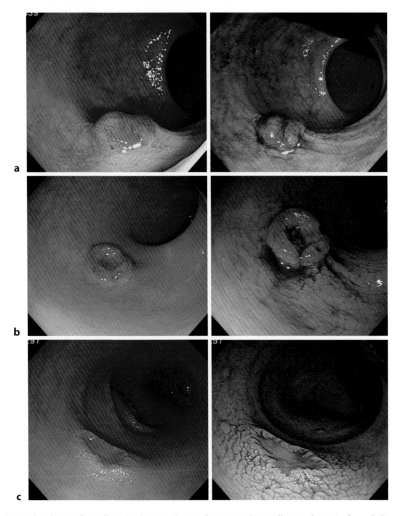

Fig. 3. Endoscopic views of small and minute colorectal cancers that ordinary views (**a**, **b**, **c**, *left*) and dye spraying views (**a**, **b**, **c**, *right*)

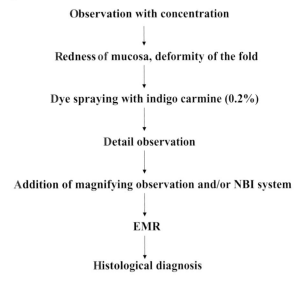

Fig. 4. Diagnostic protocol for small and minute colorectal cancers. *NBI*, narrow band imaging; *EMR*, endoscopic mucosal resection

References

1. O'Brien MJ, Winawer SJ, Zauber AG, et al (1990) The national polyp study: patient and polyp characteristics associated with high grade dysplasia in colorectal adenomas. Gastroenterology 98:371–379
2. Vatn MH, Stalsberg H (1982) The prevalence of polyps of the large intestine in Oslo; an autopsy study. Cancer 82 49:819–825.
3. Axelrad AM, Fleischer DE, Geller AJ, et al (1996) High-resolution chromoendoscopy for the diagnosis of diminutive colon polyps; implications for colon cancer screening. Gastroenterology 110:1253–1258
4. Muto T, Kamiya J, Sawada T, et al (1985) Small "flat adenoma" of the large bowel with special reference to its clinicopathologic features. Dig Colon Rectum 28:847–851
5. Kudo S, Tamura S, Hirota S, et al (1995) The problem of de novo colorectal carcinoma. Eur J Cancer 31:1118–1120
6. Minamoto T, Sawaguchi K, Ohta T, et al (1994) Superficial-type adenoma and adenocarcinomas of the colon and rectum; a comparative morphological study. Gastroenterology 106:1436–1443
7. Nakajima T, Saito Y, Matsuda T, et al (2007) Minute depressed-type submucosal invasive cancer 5 mm in diameter with intermediate lymph-node metastasis: report of a case. Dis Colon Rectum 50:677–681
8. Winawer SJ, Fletcher RH, Miller L, et al (1997) Colorectal cancer screening: clinical guidelines and rationale. Gastroenterology 112:594–642
9. Kudo S, Hirota S, Nakajima T, et al (1994) Colorectal tumors and pit pattern. J Clin Pathol 47:880–885
10. Sano Y, Horimatsu T, Ki FU, et al (2006) Magnifying observation of microvascular architecture of colorectal lesion using a narrow band imaging system. Dig Endosc 18:s44–s51
11. Tsuda S, Kikuchi Y (1999) Diagnostic ability of conventional endoscopy in colorectal neoplasms. Stomach Intestine 34:1623–1633

Magnifying Endoscopy with Narrow Band Imaging for Diagnosis of Early Colorectal Cancer

Naoyuki Uragami

Introduction

Narrow band imaging (NBI) was developed by Gono et al. (1) and has been applied widely for the diagnosis of cancer by gastrointestinal endoscopy. In cases of colorectal tumors, in particular, a number of reports have demonstrated the potential utility of NBI for: 1) detecting lesions at screening colonoscopy (2, 3); 2) qualitative diagnosis based on pit patterns and tumor surface vessels (4–8); and 3) predicting invasion depth. No dye is used for the NBI observation, and digital NBI images (image-enhanced endoscopy) can be obtained easily at the touch of a button on the electronic endoscope. With no requirement for troublesome procedures such as dye spraying and rinsing of the lesion, NBI has been accepted with ease by endoscopists worldwide.

A variety of studies (2, 3) have investigated the utility of NBI for colorectal cancer screening. However, this NBI system remains controversial because fluid remaining in the bowel appears reddish, visibility becomes low in cases of poor bowel preparation, and NBI images appear differently from those obtained with conventional white-light endoscopy.

Given the capability of NBI for pit pattern diagnosis without dye spraying (5), magnifying endoscopy with NBI has been employed extensively. However, the enabling NBI system, with its high-contrast images reflecting hemoglobin's strong absorption of narrow bandwidth light in blood vessels, will likely come to be used for qualitative diagnosis based on vascular patterns and for predicting tumor invasion depth (Table 1, Figs 1, 2, 3).

Table 1. Classification of vascular patterns

Unclear pattern
Regular pattern
Meshed type (fine net)
Short spiral
Long spiral
Irregular pattern
Thick, coarse vessel
Spotted

Fujita, Takahashi (Eds.), *Gastrointestinal Cancer Atlas for Endoscopic Therapy*, DOI: 10.1007/978-4-431-88166-7_10
© Springer

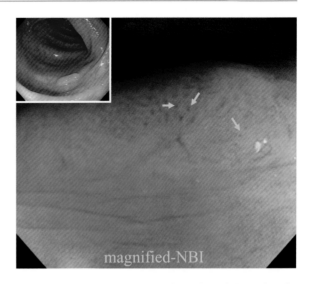

Fig. 1. *Unclear patterns*: We cannot recognize vascular on the surface of the lesion using the magnified NBI system. The unclear patterns have been reported previously as a nonneoplastic lesion. This was a hyperplastic polyp

The results of our experience with these diagnostic methods are as follows. Among 17500 consecutive patients who underwent colonoscopy at the Cancer Institute Hospital of the Japanese Foundation for Cancer Research (JFCR) between January 2004 and August 2007, a total of 1640 colorectal lesions were observed using the NBI system with an Olympus magnifying endoscope (magnified NBI). The vascular patterns visualized by magnified NBI were classified and then compared to the histopathological diagnosis of cancer invasion. We classified three vascular patterns: unclear patterns, regular patterns (meshed, short spiral, long spiral pattern), and irregular patterns (thick vascular and spotted). The histopathological diagnoses were nonneoplasm in 261 lesions, adenoma in 1218 lesions, Ca in situ (M) in 84 lesions, submucosal slight invasion (SM-sl) in 18 lesions, and submucosal massive invasion (SM-m) in 59 lesions. The vascular patterns determined by magnified NBI were unclear in 177 lesions, regular in 1399 lesions, and irregular in 64 lesions. Of the 177 lesions showing unclear vascular patterns on magnified NBI, 146 (82%) were found to be nonneoplasms based on their histopathology. In total, 88 of 102 (86%) M and SM-sl lesions showed regular vascular patterns, whereas 50 of 59 (85%) SM-m lesions showed irregular vascular patterns (Tables 2 and 3).

The vascular pattern shown on magnified NBI is associated with the depth of cancer invasion and surface vascularity in colorectal lesions. An irregular vascular pattern is a useful indication of the need for surgical treatment of early colorectal cancer.

The NBI system allows endoscopic diagnosis without the use of dye spraying and is therefore likely to become a standard technique in the future. For large lesions, however, it is necessary to carry out chromo-endoscopy with indigo carmine staining of the lesion, where magnifying observation is required. In addition, when irregular vascularity is detected by NBI, it is necessary to carry out a pit pattern diagnosis

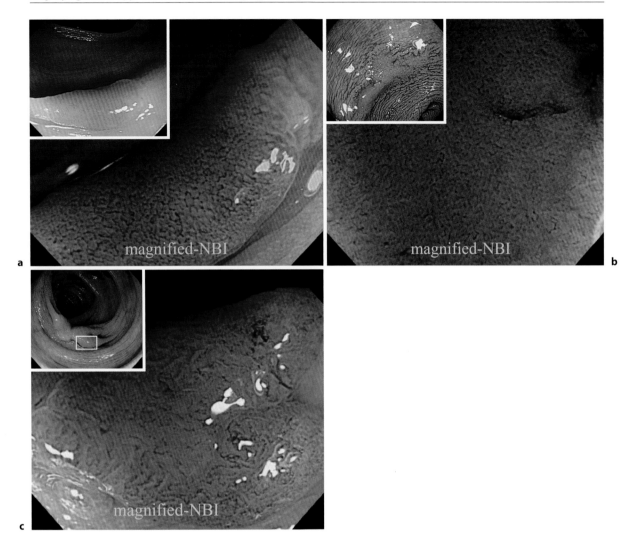

Fig. 2. *Regular vascular patterns*
a Meshed (fine network) type, one of the regular vascular patterns. The vascular patterns make a fine network on the surface. This lesion was a tubular adenoma
b Short spiral type, one of the regular vascular patterns. The lesion was a mucosal cancer
c Long spiral type, one of the regular vascular patterns. The lesion was a carcinoma with an adenoma

with crystal violet staining. Although pit patterns can be observed by NBI, this system was originally developed to enhance visualization of the vasculature. Therefore, it is important to use NBI based on its original intention and diagnostic capabilities—that is, qualitative diagnosis based on tumor surface vessels and the prediction of tumor invasion depth.

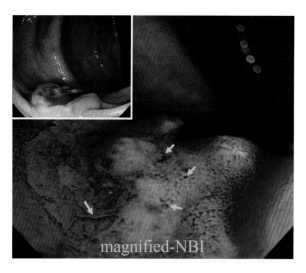

Fig. 3. *Irregular vascular pattern*: Spotted vascularity with a thick, coarse vessel on the surface. The lesion was found at surgery to be invasive adenocarcinoma

Table 2. Vascularity and depth of invasion

Invasion	Unclear pattern	Regular patterns			Irregular pattern	Total
		Meshed	Short spiral	Long spiral		
Non	146	85	27	3	0	261
Ad	31	601	481	105	0	1218
M	0	9	28	39	8	84
SM 1	0	2	6	4	6	18
SM 2	0	2	2	5	50	59
Total	177	699	544	156	64	1640

Non, nonneoplasm; Ad, adenoma; M, mucosal cancer; SM sl, sm slight invasion; SM m, sm massive invasion
Results are the number of lesions

Table 3. Possibility of analyzing vascular patterns

Invasion	Unclear pattern (%)	Regular patterns (%)			Irregular pattern
		Meshed	Short spiral	Long spiral	
Non	82	12	5	2	0
Ad	18	86	88	67	0
M	0	1	5	25	13
SM sl	0	0.3	1.1	3	9
SM m	0	0.3	0.4	3	78

References

1. Gono K, Obi T, Yamaguchi M, et al (2004) Appearance of enhanced tissue features in narrow-band endoscopic imaging. J Biomed Opt 9:568–577
2. Adler A, Pohl H, Papanikolaou IS, et al (2008) A prospective randomised study on narrow-band imaging versus conventional colonoscopy for adenoma detection: does narrow-band imaging induce a learning effect? Gut 57:59–64
3. Inoue T, Murano M, Murano N, et al (2008) Comparative study of conventional colonoscopy and pan-colonic narrow-band imaging system in the detection of neoplastic colonic polyps: a randomized, controlled trial. J Gastroenterol 43:45–50
4. Machida H, Sano Y, Hamamoto Y, et al (2004) Narrow-band imaging in the diagnosis of colorectal mucosal lesions: a pilot study. Endoscopy 36:1094–1098
5. Su MY, Hsu CM, Ho YP, et al (2006) Comparative study of conventional colonoscopy, chromoendoscopy, and narrow-band imaging systems in differential diagnosis of neoplastic and nonneoplastic colonic polyps. Am J Gastroenterol 101:2711–2716
6. Hirata M, Tanaka S, Oka S, et al (2007) Evaluation of microvessels in colorectal tumors by narrow band imaging magnification. Gastrointest Endosc 66:945–952
7. Chiu HM, Chang CY, Chen CC, et al (2007) A prospective comparative study of narrow-band imaging, chromoendoscopy, and conventional colonoscopy in the diagnosis of colorectal neoplasia. Gut 56:373–379
8. Tischendorf JJ, Wasmuth HE, Koch A, et al (2007) Value of magnifying chromoendoscopy and narrow band imaging (NBI) in classifying colorectal polyps: a prospective controlled study. Endoscopy 39:1092–1096

Case 1

70-year-old man early colon cancer, ascending, type 0-IIc, 10 mm well-differentiated adenocarcinoma.

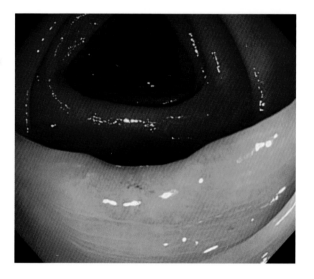

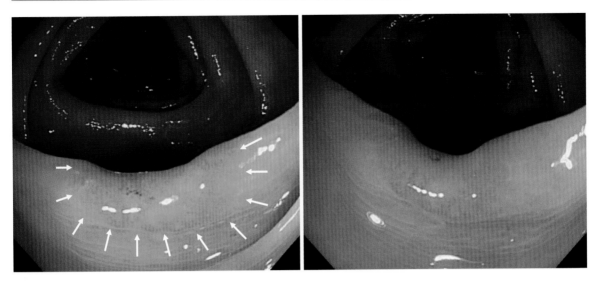

Fig. 1. Endoscopic diagnosis and findings
Routine observation: A slightly reddish, ill-demarcated, depressed lesion (*arrows*) is apparent. No fold convergence, erosion, or ulceration was observed at the depression. After slight deflation, the depression became more evident, but no marginal elevation or fold convergence was observed

Diagnostic Points:

Color changes were mild, and detection of the lesion was difficult. Observation of fold irregularity under slightly deflated conditions was the key to detecting the lesion.

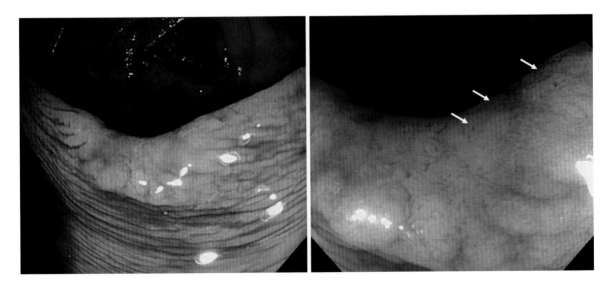

Fig. 2. *Indigo carmine spraying*: Dye spraying visualized the margin of the lesion more clearly. The surface of the depression was a little rough, but no irregularity was observed
Magnifying observation: Magnification revealed scattered type III$_s$ pits (*arrows*) at the center of the depression, although some areas remained unclear

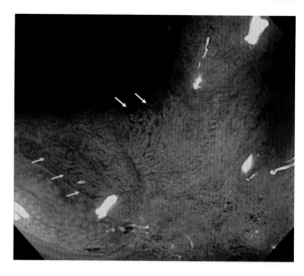

Fig. 3. *NBI*: Magnifying narrow band imaging (NBI) showed slightly larger blood vessels at the center (*white arrows*). A vascular network pattern, including other blood vessels (*yellow arrows*), was observed

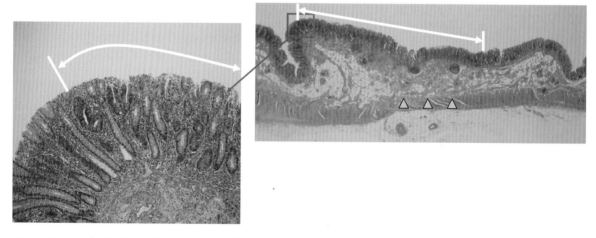

Fig. 4. *Pathological findings*: The lesion was localized to the area indicated by the *arrows*, and there was no difference in height between the normal and cancerous crypts. Fibrosis was observed at the submucosal layer (*arrowheads*), which was suspected to be the cause of the positive non-lifting sign
Histology: well-differentiated adenocarcinoma, depth pM, ly0, v0

Case 2

67-year-old man early rectal cancer, lower posterior rectum, type 0-IIa+IIc, 10 mm cancer with adenoma.

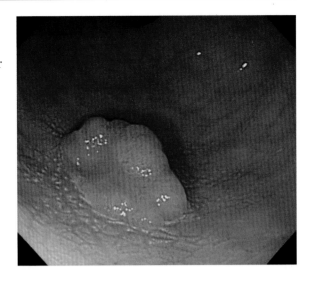

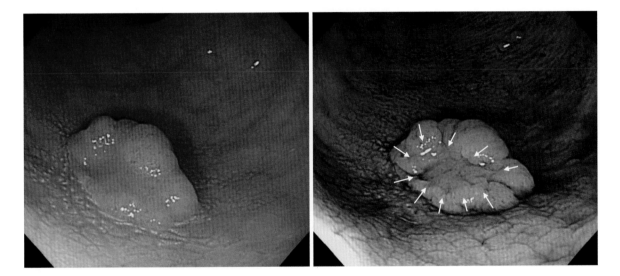

Fig. 1. Endoscopic diagnosis and findings
Routine observation: A type Is+IIc lesion, 10 mm in diameter, with peripheral white patches
Indigo carmine spraying: Dye spraying more clearly visualized the depression with slightly reddish changes (*arrows*)

Diagnostic Points:

Early cancer was suspected based on the presence of peripheral white patches, and a depression was confirmed after indigo carmine spraying.

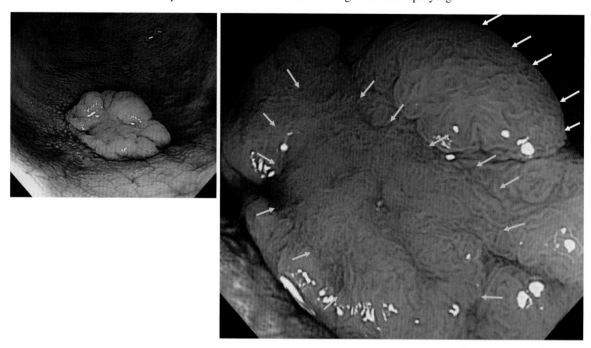

Fig. 2. *Indigo carmine spraying (magnified)*: Magnifying observation with indigo carmine spraying revealed type III_L pits at the marginal elevation (*white arrows*) and the type V_I pit pattern at the depression (*yellow arrows*)

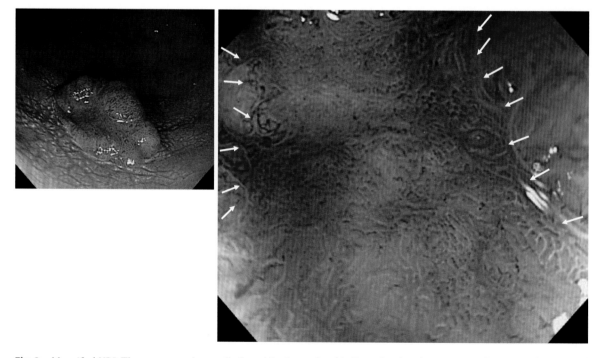

Fig. 3. *Magnified NBI*: There were no abnormally large blood vessels with disruption, but there was a surface network pattern of blood vessels on the depressed surface (*white arrows*)

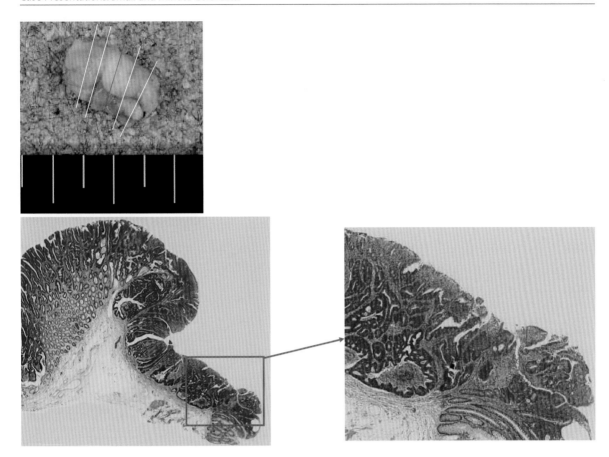

Fig. 4. Picture of resection specimen.
Pathological findings: Well-differentiated adenocarcinoma was present exactly at the depression
Histology: Well-differentiated adenocarcinoma (cancer with adenoma), depth pM, ly0, v0

Case 3

68-year-old man early rectal cancer, upper rectum, type 0-Isp, 10 mm cancer with adenoma.

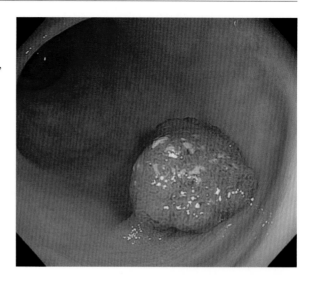

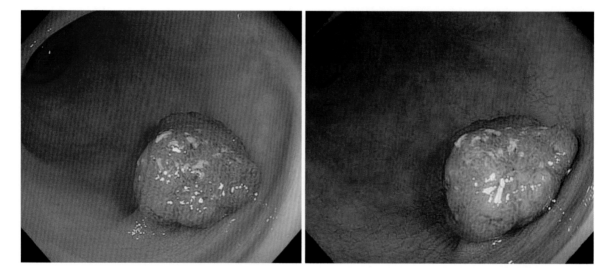

Fig. 1. Endoscopic diagnosis and findings

Routine observation: A reddish type Isp lesion accompanied by mild fold irregularity

Indigo carmine spraying: Dye spraying revealed that the depressed area at the center seemed to be elevated compared with the margin, and the surface of the elevated area was rough

Diagnostic Points:

There were mild heterogeneous color changes and a gap in height at the margin after indigo carmine spraying. Dye spraying revealed that the depression had elevated as the tumor grew.

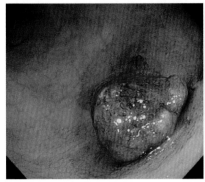
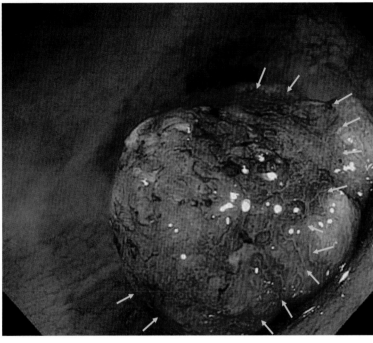

Fig. 2. *Crystal violet staining*: Magnifying observation after crystal violet staining revealed the type V_N pit pattern on the elevated area (*yellow arrows*)

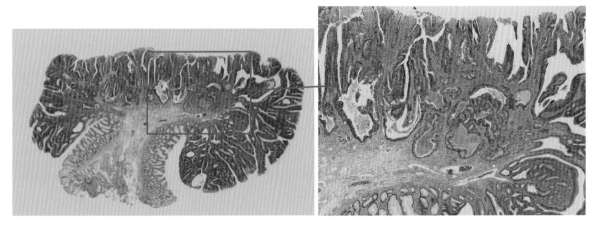

Fig. 3. *Pathological findings*: Well-differentiated adenocarcinoma was present exactly at the depression. The margin showed adenoma components
Histology: well-differentiated adenocarcinoma (cancer with adenoma), depth pSM (2200 μm), ly1, v0

Case 4

58-year-old woman early colon cancer, sigmoid, type 0-Is, 10 mm moderately differentiated adenocarcinoma.

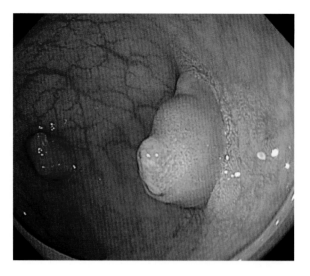

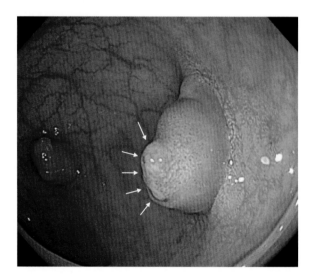

Fig. 1. Endoscopic diagnosis and findings

Routine observation: An elevated lesion, 10 mm in diameter, was observed in the sigmoid colon about 27 cm from the AV (Anal Verge). The color was mildly reddish and homogeneous. White patches were observed at the periphery. The tumor had an even higher elevation on the top (*arrows*), with fullness. Mobility was somewhat poor when the root of the tumor was pushed by the forceps

Diagnostic Points:

In this case, the lesion was detected by total colonoscopy performed as the secondary medical investigation of the positive immunological fecal occult blood test. Despite the small size, an elevated lesion with further elevation on the top is a finding suggestive of infiltration to the submucosal (SM) layer. Laparoscopic sigmoidectomy was performed.

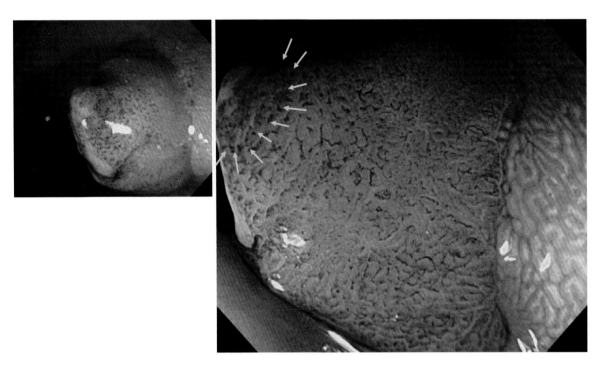

Fig. 2. *Magnified NBI*: A network pattern of blood vessels on the surface was revealed, except at the top of the lesion, where large irregular, disrupted blood vessels were visualized (*yellow arrows*)

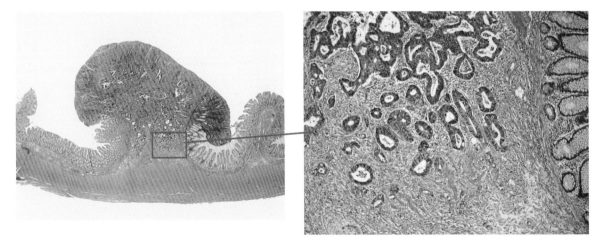

Fig. 3. *Pathological findings*: The surface structure of the 10 × 10 mm tumor was preserved, but the tumor showed poorer differentiation in the deep part; infiltration into the SM layer was also observed. (H&E × 200)
Histology: type Is moderately differentiated adenocarcinoma, ly2, v0, pN0 (0/15)

Case 5

56-year-old man early colon cancer, sigmoid, type 0-IIa+IIc, 10 mm moderately differentiated adenocarcinoma.

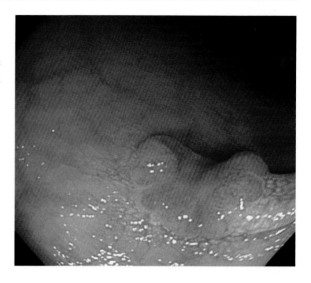

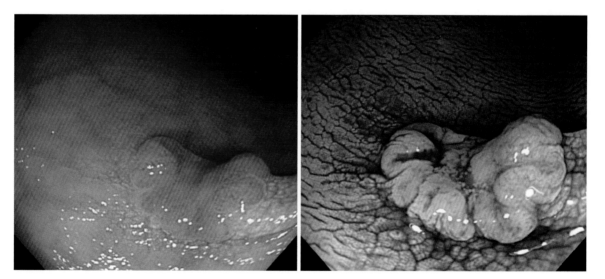

Fig. 1. Endoscopic diagnosis and findings
Routine observation: A type IIa+IIc lesion, 10 mm in diameter, was observed in the sigmoid colon 20 cm from the AV. Pushing with forceps showed slightly poor mobility, and there were no morphological changes upon air inflation/deflation
Indigo carmine spraying: Dye spraying more clearly visualized the depression

Diagnostic Points:

The lesion was detected by total colonoscopy performed secondary to a positive immunological fecal occult blood test. The depression, although small, was apparent. Observations of no morphological changes in the depressed surface upon air inflation/deflation and the irregular structure of the depressed surface were the keys to diagnosis. Laparoscopic sigmoidectomy was carried out.

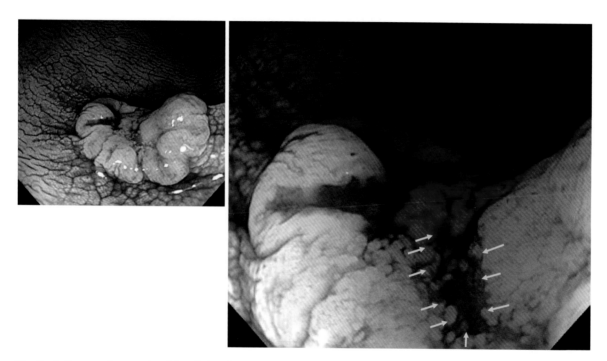

Fig. 2. *Indigo carmine spraying*: Magnifying observation with indigo carmine spraying revealed normal pits at the margin of the elevation and destroyed pits on the depressed surface (*yellow arrows*)

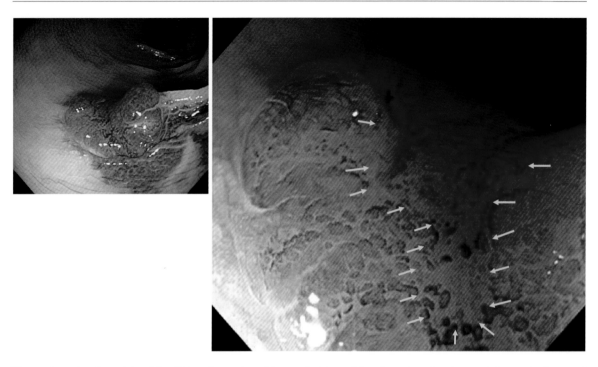

Fig. 3. *Crystal violet staining*: Magnifying observation with crystal violet staining showed patchy pits remaining on the depressed surface and type V_N pits on the depressed surface (*yellow arrows*)

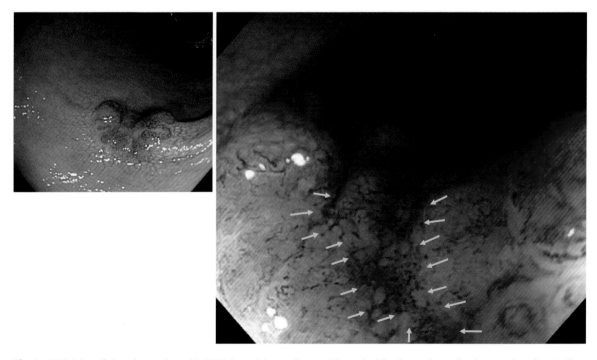

Fig. 4. *NBI*: Magnifying observation with NBI showed large, disrupted irregular blood vessels on the depressed surface (*yellow arrows*)

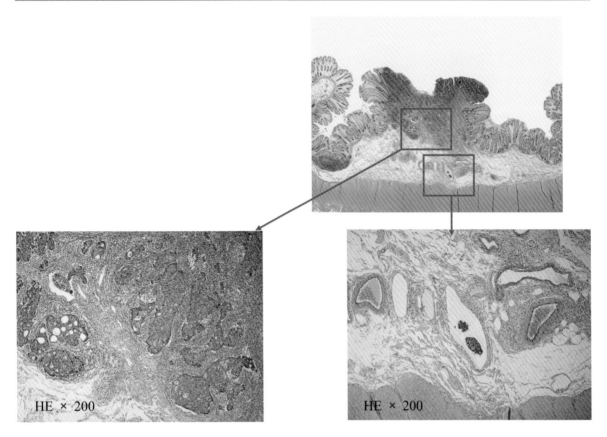

Fig. 5. *Pathological findings*: The advancing front showed an invasion tendency with poorer differentiation. Severe vascular infiltration was also observed

Histology: 10 mm; type IIa+IIc, moderately differentiated adenocarcinoma, pSM (2230 μm), ly2, v0, pN0 (0/12)

Case 6

64-year-old man early colon cancer, sigmoid, type 0-Isp, 10 mm well-differentiated adenocarcinoma.

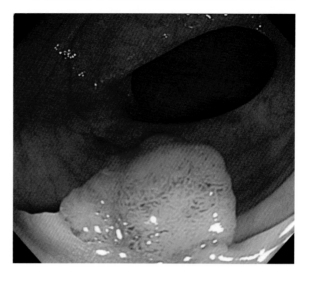

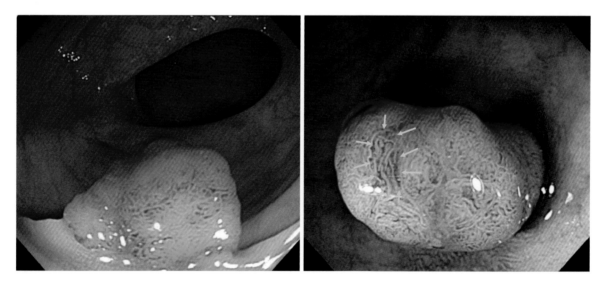

Fig. 1. Endoscopic diagnosis and findings
Routine observation: A type Isp polyp, 10 mm in diameter, was observed in the sigmoid colon. Its color was heterogeneous, and it exhibited peripheral white patches
Indigo carmine spraying: Dye spraying revealed type III$_L$ and IV pits (*yellow arrows*)

Diagnostic Points:

The lesion was detected by total colonoscopy following a positive fecal occult blood test. Endoscopic mucosal resection (EMR) was carried out.

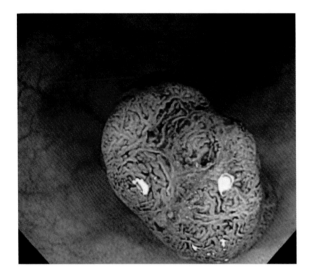

Fig. 2. *NBI*: A vascular network pattern of superficial blood vessels was visualized all over the tumor

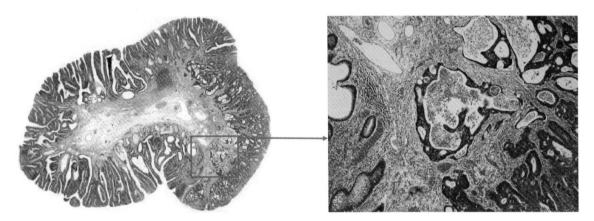

Fig. 3. *Pathological findings*: Tubular adenoma with moderate atypia
Histology: adenocarcinoma, well-to moderately differentiated, depth pSM1, ly0, v0

Case 7

74-year-old woman early colon cancer, transverse, type 0-IIa, 10 mm well-differentiated adenocarcinoma.

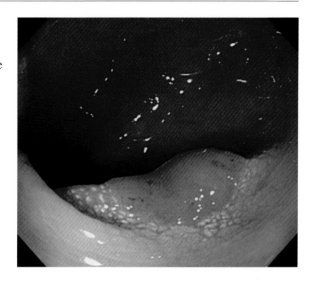

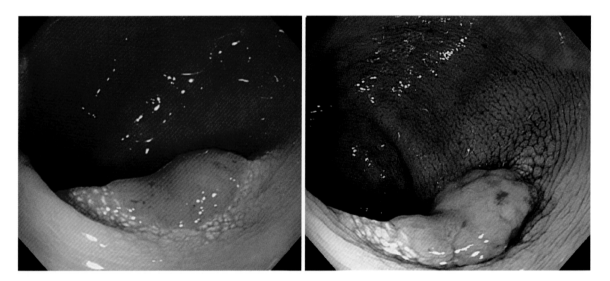

Fig. 1. Endoscopic diagnosis and findings
Routine observation: A reddish, flat-elevated lesion with peripheral white patches was observed in the transverse colon
Indigo carmine spraying: Dye spraying showed a slightly depressed area at the center of the tumor

Diagnostic Points:

A superficial tumor with peripheral white patches was seen. Magnified visualization showed differing results in that pit patterns were types IIIs and V_I after indigo carmine spraying and crystal violet staining, respectively. However, given only the mild irregularity of the type V_I pits, EMR was performed based on the suspicion of mucosal cancer.

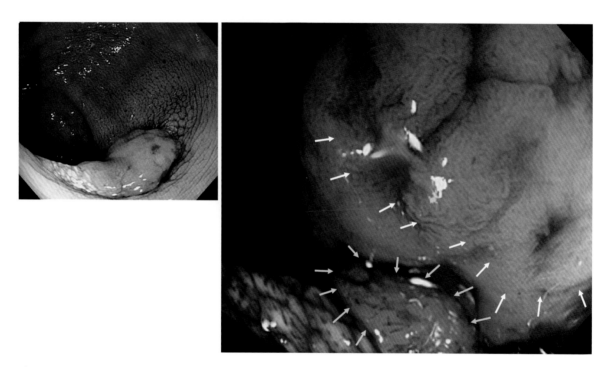

Fig. 2. *Indigo carmine spraying*: Magnifying observation after indigo carmine spraying showed type III_L pits at the margin (*white arrows*) and type V_I pits at the depression (*yellow arrows*)

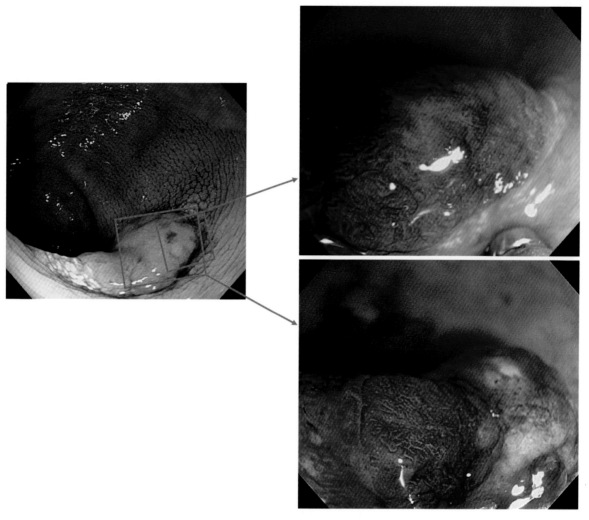

Fig. 3. *Crystal violet staining*: Magnifying observation with crystal violet staining revealed type V_I pits in the area where type III_L pits were observed after indigo carmine spraying. Type V_I pits were observed all over the tumor

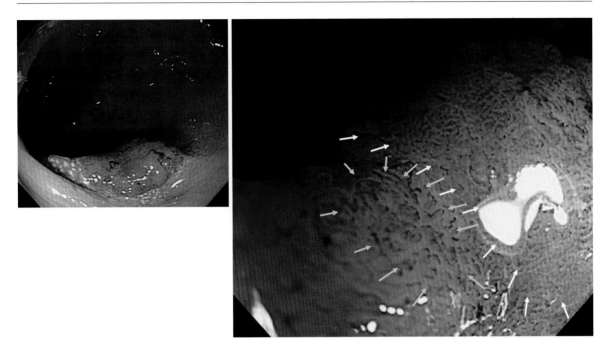

Fig. 4. *NBI*: Magnifying NBI showed a vascular network pattern of the superficial blood vessels at the margin (*white arrows*) and severely irregular blood vessels at the boundary of the depression (*yellow arrows*)

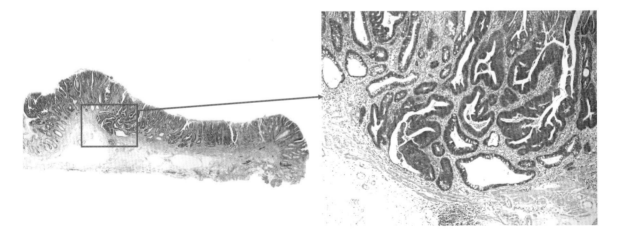

Fig. 5. *Pathological findings*: Infiltration into the muscularis mucosae was observed at the depression. Thin-sliced specimens revealed that cancer partially infiltrated the muscularis mucosae. (H&E × 400)
Histology: well-differentiated adenocarcinoma, depth pM, ly–, v–

Case 8

77-year-old woman early colon cancer, transverse, type 0-IIa, 8 mm well-differentiated adenocarcinoma.

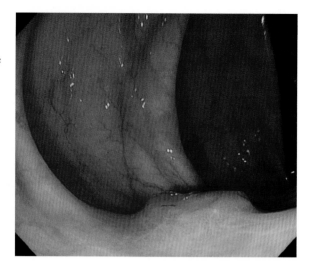

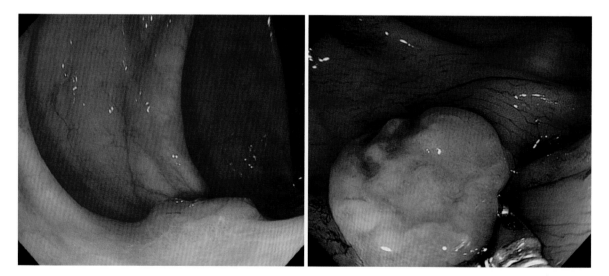

Fig. 1. Endoscopic diagnosis and findings

Routine observation: A flat-elevated lesion, 8 mm in diameter, was observed in the transverse colon. The margin of the elevation was covered with normal mucosa, and the surface of the tumor was relatively firm

Indigo carmine spraying: Dye spraying showed a depression with irregularity on the surface of the lesion

Diagnostic Points:

A small lesion was detected by total colonoscopy following a positive fecal occult blood test. This case is rare in that only type V_N pits were observed at the depression, and the marginal elevation was covered by normal mucosa.

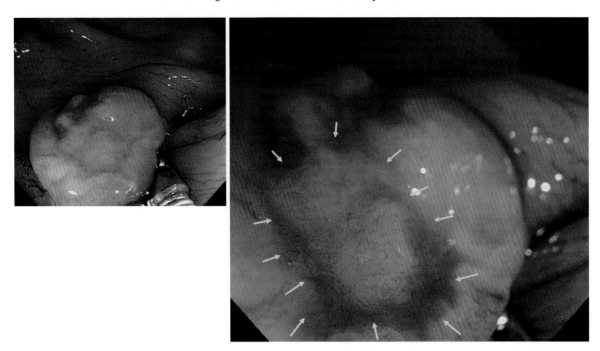

Fig. 2. *Indigo carmine spraying*: Magnified visualization after indigo carmine spraying revealed no pit patterns at the depression (*yellow arrows*)

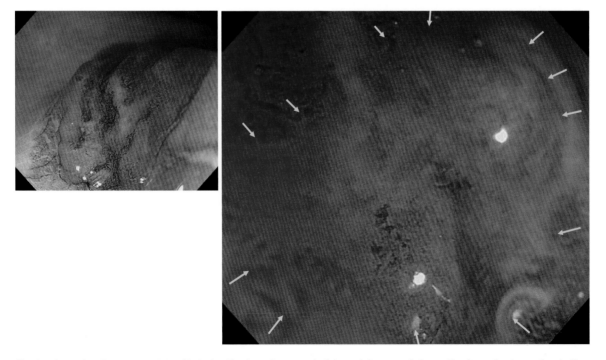

Fig. 3. *Crystal violet staining*: Magnified visualization after crystal violet staining revealed type V_N pits at the depression (*yellow arrows*)

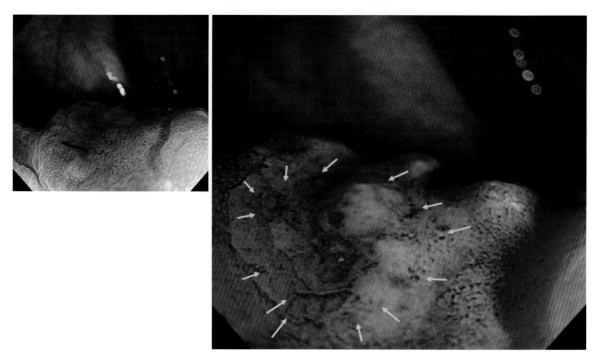

Fig. 4. *NBI*: Magnified NBI revealed that superficial blood vessels did not form a vascular network at the depression (*yellow arrows*)

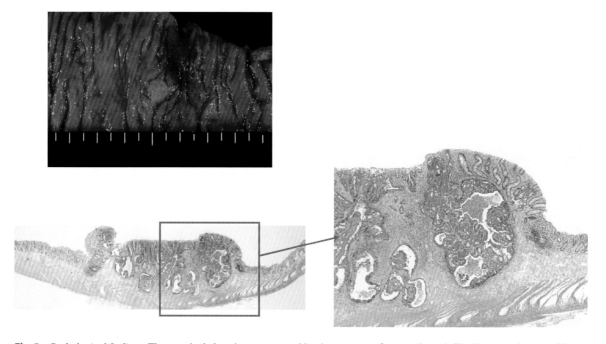

Fig. 5. *Pathological findings*: The marginal elevation was created by the pressure of cancer tissue infiltrating the submucosal layer. Given the lack of adenoma components, it was diagnosed as de novo-type early invasive cancer. (H&E × 200)
Histology: well-differentiated adenocarcinoma, depth pSM3, ly−, v−

Index